Practitioner's Guide to
Behavioral Problems in Children

Practitioner's Guide to Behavioral Problems in Children

Glen P. Aylward

Southern Illinois University School of Medicine
Springfield, Illinois

KLUWER ACADEMIC / PLENUM PUBLISHERS
New York, Boston, Dordrecht, London, Moscow

Library of Congress Cataloging-in-Publication Data

Aylward, Glen P.
    Practitioner's guide to behavioral problems in children / by Glen P. Aylward.
        p. cm.
    Includes bibliographical references and index.
    ISBN 0-306-47740-8
        1. Problem children–Behavior modification. 2. Behavior disorders in children. I. Title.

HQ773.A95 2003

649'.64–dc21   2003044718

ISBN 0-306-47740-8

© 2003 Kluwer Academic/Plenum Publishers, New York
233 Spring Street, New York, New York 10013

http://www.wkap.nl

10 9 8 7 6 5 4 3 2 1

A C.I.P. record for this book is available from the Library of Congress.

Permissions for books published in Europe: *permissions@wkap.nl*
Permissions for books published in the United States of America: *permissions@wkap.com*

Printed in the United States of America.

To Deborah for your support, and to Shawn, Megan, Brandon and Mason for the opportunity to experience on-the-job training, love and thanks.

GPA

Preface

Over the last 25 years of clinical practice, I have been impressed with a paradox, namely, the uniqueness in each child, in contrast to the frequent commonalities found in the development of behavioral problems. I have also been duly impressed with the resilience of children and their families, and the impact that provision of knowledge regarding development and behavior can have on facilitating this resilience. Guidance provided by the practitioner to caretakers can have a tremendous influence in altering the course of a behavioral concern, particularly if this guidance is provided early in the evolution of the potential problem, and is directed toward skill development in the parents. Moreover, if parents can be provided with basic principles of behavior, and are able to self-monitor their reactions to the behaviors of their child, the likelihood of a positive outcome is enhanced.

With these considerations in mind, the purpose of this book is two-fold. First, it provides a quick reference for the practitioner regarding parenting, child development, and conceptualizing, identifying, and treating behavioral concerns. The text is geared to be a practical, quick read, which the practitioner can use in anticipatory guidance or first-tier interventions. The second purpose is to provide a reference for parents. More specifically, clinicians may recommend the book to parents as a so-called bibliotherapeutic aid, either to be read independently or used in conjunction with an intervention program provided by the practitioner.

The book is not designed to be highly detailed; rather, it is broad-based and provides a model or framework from which to approach behavioral problems. As a result, the number of references has purposefully been kept to a minimum.

I am indebted to my young patients and their families for providing me with the opportunity over the years to work with them and learn together how to address behavioral concerns. I am also grateful to my editor, Siiri Lelumees, for her patience and flexibility during the preparation of this book. I truly hope this book might, in some small way, have a positive influence in improving the life of a child and his family, either directly or indirectly. If so, this effort has been worthwhile.

Contents

                Summary. 121

Chapter 9   **Quick Reference: Signs, Reinforcements,**
            Techniques, and Considerations 123
                Aggression (Young Child) 123
                Aggression (Older Child) 124
                Argumentativeness 125
                Bedwetting 126
                Excessive Fears 127
                Food Refusal 127
                Masturbatory Behavior 128
                Mutism 129
                Noncompliance 130
                Refusal to Take Medication 131
                School Behavioral Problem 131
                School Refusal 132
                Separation Issue 133
                Sibling Conflict 134
                Sleep Problem 135
                Soiling 136
                Somatic Concerns 137
                Temper Tantrums 137
                Thumbsucking 138
                Whining 139

Chapter 10 **Summary and Musings 141**

            References 147

            Index 153

Practitioner's Guide to Behavioral Problems in Children

Chapter 1

Introduction

It is estimated that 13%–22% of the pediatric population has some type of behavioral or emotional problem. The prevalence is doubled in lower socioeconomic status households. In fact, 70% to 80% of parents have a behavioral concern when they visit their child's physician for routine or acute care and the vast majority will not bring these concerns up unless they are solicited. It is estimated that 90% of mothers of 2- to 4-year-old children have "some" concern about their child's behavior; 20% of mothers of 4-year olds have significant concerns. Unfortunately, primary care physicians (PCPs) have not been especially effective in detecting such problems, the sensitivity rate being 4%–7%. Interestingly, the strongest predictor of whether PCPs will detect a given behavioral problem is familiarity with the patient, or, more specifically, continuity of care (Kelleher et al., 1997; Kelleher & Wolraich, 1996). Without doubt, this becomes increasingly difficult in today's healthcare environment.

PCPs typically are the point of access for children who manifest behavioral or emotional problems, as pediatricians and family practitioners handle three quarters of all office-based visits per year. Therefore, these physicians have the most routine contact with children during these years, have established trust and familiarity with the family, and, in a more pragmatic vein, often are required by many insurance plans to make a determination as to the appropriateness of a referral to psychologists or other mental health professionals. Moreover, most parents prefer to obtain an initial impression about the problematic behavior and suggestions regarding intervention from their child's physician, versus simply going to the yellow pages to locate a mental health professional (Costello, 1986; Costello & Edelbrock, 1985). On average, of a hypothetical five children who display a behavioral or emotional concern, one will not receive any intervention, one will be seen by a mental health professional, and the remaining three will be treated solely by the PCP.

Practitioners and parents are routinely faced with the question whether a behavior is normal, abnormal, or somewhere in between. This determination is important, as it will drive what is said and done about the behavior. In other words, it is often difficult to determine whether a behavior is typical or atypical because of the impreciseness of any classification scheme. There simply is no clear-cut one or two standard deviations below the mean cutoff or any 'gold standard' that can be used as a benchmark for many behavioral concerns. For example, if there is a question about physical growth, growth curves can be used for verification. Lab values can help determine whether a medical problem should be treated or not. Age norms are employed when questions about development arise, and occupation and level of education help to quantify socioeconomic status. Unfortunately, there is no such measurement that can be applied in the case of a "subclinical" behavioral concern.

Similarly, how we describe a behavior may determine what is done about it, with descriptions of the same behaviors potentially ranging from benign to problematic. For example, a child with a high activity level may be described as overly active, bouncy, or hyperactive. The child who does not seek out social interaction may be considered independent, a loner, or socially maladjusted. Finally, a noncompliant youngster could be called strong-willed, ornery, or oppositional/defiant. The descriptor that is selected depends on the child's age, severity of behavior, and the relationship that the person who assigns the descriptor has with the child.

Such "labeling" is important for several reasons. Once assigned, a label is difficult to remove. In fact, this is one reason why the non-categorical term, "developmental delay," is often used in order to obtain intervention services for young children. Conversely, assigning a benign term such as "strong-willed" instead of a more accurate diagnosis of oppositional/ defiant disorder may not necessarily be in the child's best interests, because the untreated Oppositional Defiant Disorders (ODD) most likely would put the child out of synchrony with peers and have a negative impact on his self-concept and self-esteem.

BEHAVIORAL PROBLEMS IN INFANTS AND YOUNG CHILDREN

Behavioral problems in infants and young children group into the six categories indicated below. While some of the behavioral categories fall into the broad band syndromes of undercontrolled, externalizing behaviors or overcontrolled, internalizing behaviors, others do not (Aylward, 1992).

1. Problems of daily routines (food refusal, bedtime, toilet training)

2. Aggressive-resistant behavior (negativism, temper tantrums, aggressiveness toward siblings or peers)
3. Overdependent/withdrawing behavior (demanding, separation upset, clinging, whining, excessive fearfulness)
4. Hyperactivity/excessive restlessness
5. Undesirable habits (night awakening, thumb sucking, nail biting, masturbation)
6. Developmental variations

Many of the problems faced by PCPs are not of the severity to warrant a diagnosis based on the *Diagnostic and Statistical Manual of Mental Disorders (DSM-IV*; American Psychiatric Association, 1994), either due to the magnitude of the problem or age of the child. Nonetheless, these "subclinical" or "subthreshold" problems cause distress for the family and potentially may interfere with the child's development. Early detection and treatment prevents these behaviors from developing into more severe problems that are more disruptive, cause increased suffering for the child and family, and require more costly treatment. For example, the child who bites, the excessive whiner, the child who displays idiosyncratic toileting behaviors, or the preschooler who demonstrates excessive temper tantrums does not necessarily meet the diagnostic criteria necessary for a true DSM-IV diagnosis, yet intervention is necessary.

DIAGNOSTIC AND STATISTICAL MANUAL-PRIMARY CARE (DSM-PC)

To this end, the *Diagnostic and Statistical Manual-Primary Care, Child and Adolescent Version (DSM-PC*; Wolraich, Felice, & Drotar, 1996) was developed. This text was designed to address recognition, classification, and diagnostic issues for the PCP; however, two important assumptions are made in the *DSM-PC* that are particularly pertinent to the content of this book. First, the *environment* of the child will have a major impact or influence on his or her behavior and mental health. Second, symptoms or behaviors that children demonstrate vary along a *spectrum*, ranging from normal developmental variations, to problems, to true disorders. This latter assumption has important ramifications in terms of description of the disorder, intervention, and portraying the severity for parents. Essentially it is rare that a behavioral concern is simply a yes/no proposition, as these concerns vary in terms of degree and nature. Even with more severe developmental disorders such as autism, Tourettes, or an attention deficit hyperactivity disorder, the child may fit a yes/no format in terms of having the disorder, but the disorder itself is on a continuum ranging from mild to moderate to severe. This gradation will influence treatment choices and prognosis.

According to the *DSM-PC*, the three points on the diagnostic spectrum are:

- *Developmental variation:* such behavior is a concern, but is still within the range of expected behaviors for a child of a given age. For example, many 4-year-olds are brought to their PCPs because of a suspected attention deficit hyperactivity disorder. A large number of the symptoms are displayed simply by virtue of being 4-years of age; even if the behaviors meet the criteria for ADHD found in the *DSM-IV*, fully one-third of the 4-year-old children will not have that diagnosis 6 months later. These types of behaviors can be adequately addressed by guidance and counseling.
- *Problem:* this involves a behavioral concern that is further along the spectrum, and is of sufficient magnitude so as to disrupt the child's interactions and functioning in: (a) the family, (b) school, and/or (c) peer interactions. However, the severity or type of problem does not warrant the diagnosis of a mental disorder. Excessive aggressiveness, refusal to toilet at age 4, or social withdrawal are examples. Such problems may be handled by the PCP, although psychologists, social workers, or other mental health specialists often will also provide treatment.
- *Disorder:* This behavioral concern meets *DSM-IV* criteria for an actual disorder. While some disorders such as enuresis, encopresis, a tic disorder, or even ADHD (without comorbid conditions) may be addressed adequately by the PCP, the services of a psychologist, child psychiatrist, developmental/behavioral pediatrician, or other professionals often are needed.

To summarize this concept, a behavioral concern should be considered to lie somewhere on a diagnostic spectrum, the two anchor points being a benign normal developmental variation and a more debilitating disorder, with the "problem" category falling at the midpoint. To help determine where on the spectrum a behavioral concern lies, it is necessary to consider: (a) whether the behavior is typical given the child's age, and (b) where on the continuum of severity the behavioral concern falls, namely, *mild* (minimal negative developmental/functional impact), *moderate* (some developmental/functional impairment), and *severe* (serious developmental/functional dysfunction and difficulties). This procedure will put the problem in perspective for the parents, and also influence the type and intensity of intervention that is warranted. Unfortunately, more serious disorders are easier to identify than are subtle ones.

Age Concerns

The age of the child is also important, in terms of factors that would contribute to the behavior concern and sources of information used for diagnostic considerations and intervention. One must consider the immediate environment more strongly during infancy and the early childhood years (birth to age 5 years), and information is obtained primarily from observation of interactions and caretakers' report. How the environment reacts to the infant and preschooler will be critical in determining whether certain behavioral predispositions of the child will be maintained, attenuated, or exacerbated. For example, in the case of the anxious child, the anxiety will be exacerbated if the parents become overly sensitized and anticipatory about the child's predicted reaction, thereby going overboard in an effort to reduce stress. In so doing, the parents become more permissive and inconsistent, and inadvertently further reinforce the child's behaviors. As the child ages, there is an increasing number of environmental influences external to the family and daycare environment that may exert an effect. By school age (age 6 years to 11 or 12) the environmental circle of influences expands to include peers, school, sports, and other organized activities, in addition to the family. Therefore, while the child at this age may be more communicative with regard to the problems he or she is facing, the realm of moderating or mediating environmental influences is expanded. By adolescence, in addition to the environmental influences that affect the school age child, genetic predisposition toward psychiatric problems (e.g., depression), substance and alcohol use, sexuality, and decision-making regarding long-term issues such as career, will have an impact.

Hence the practitioner is faced with a paradox, in that with infants and children in the early childhood range, the causative factors for the behavior problem may be more limited (child predispositions and how the family/caretaker addresses these) but the information is more difficult to obtain. By school age and into adolescence, the patient may be more verbal (although not necessarily so) but the range of potential influences on a given behavioral or emotional concern expands considerably. Moreover, given that many behavioral/emotional concerns have an insidious onset and are cumulative over time, cause-effect delineations in older children and adolescents are often more tenuous.

Risk and Protective Factors

Determination of severity is subjective, but the practitioner should consider: (1) the type of symptoms the child displays (frequency, intensity, duration, amount of disruption, occurrence across situations), (2) the degree of dysfunction (impact on school, family, peers), (3) degree of "suffering" (self-esteem, impact on family functioning, social isolation), and (4) risk and protective factors (Wolraich, Felice, & Drotar, 1996). A more simplistic rule of thumb is that the practitioner needs to determine whether the behavioral concern has a negative impact on the child's ability to learn, interact socially, or causes a marked behavioral problem.

With respect to risk and protective factors, the former are negative influences that increase the child's vulnerability or draw toward non-optimal development; conversely, protective factors refer to attributes or environmental aspects that enhance the child's resilience to adverse circumstances and produce "self-righting." Risk and protective factors may be child-related or environmentally-based. Examples of child-related risk and protective factors include health (good health would be protective; a chronic medical condition would increase risk), temperament (easy child temperament is protective; a difficult child temperamental style would increase risk [see Chapter 3]), or cognitive status (average or above average intelligence would be a protective factor; borderline intelligence or mental retardation is considered a risk factor). Other child-related factors may include emotional "health," academic skills, motor abilities, language skills, and attention/activity. For a more detailed discussion of this concept, the reader is encouraged to review the *DSM-PC* (Wolraich, Felice, & Drotar, 1996).

Along the same lines, environmentally-based risk includes components such as parental competence (competent parenting being protective; poor parenting skills placing the child at risk), family resources (poverty is a definite risk factor), and stability/safety of environment. When considering the environment in terms of risk and protective factors, the practitioner is encouraged to consider three major areas:

- *Household/family:* Parent-child interaction, sibling issues, marital relationship, family dynamics, parenting skills and attitudes, physical aspects, socioeconomic status, parents' emotional and physical health.
- *School:* Teacher-child match, academics, social status, attendance, relationships with authority figures, school sports, special resource needs.
- *Peers:* friendships, contact with peers outside of school, extracurricular activities.

There is currently no specific number of risk factors that has been determined to increase the likelihood of behavioral problems. However, it is reasonable to assume that the more risk factors that are present, the greater the likelihood of such problems. It also is hypothesized that a total absence of risk or exposure to some adversity may not necessarily be as good for a child as it would initially appear. A low-grade, non-chronic, manageable amount of risk may serve as an "inoculation" in the sense that it helps the child to develop adaptive strategies and mastery. In this way, if the child is faced with adverse circumstances in the future, she would have adaptive capabilities and resiliency that might not have been developed, had she not experienced some distress in the past. Obviously, a more intense level of risk would not serve this function.

Social Status

With respect to social status, a school-aged child may be (a) *popular*, (b) *accepted* (not necessarily popular, but is able to maintain an adequate social network and level of social activity), (c) *neglected* (excluded or left out of social activities, isolated, but not picked on actively), or (d) *rejected* (isolated, bullied, picked on). Obviously, the first two statuses would be considered protective factors, while the latter two would place the child at risk. In addition, more broad, distal environmental influences include factors such as the child's neighborhood, and type of school.

Psychosocial Factors

When dealing with a child with a behavioral concern, it would be inappropriate to not consider the family and related psychosocial factors. Several authors (Costello et al., 1988; Gardiner et al., 2000; Kemper & Kelleher, 1996) have suggested that practitioners should routinely screen for psychosocial issues in parents. Depression (occurring in 12%–42% of mothers of preschoolers, depending on the sample), substance abuse (10,000,000 children currently are being raised in substance and alcohol abusing households), domestic violence (25% lifetime prevalence rate), parental history of abuse (20%–23% prevalence), and absence of social support, are significant psychosocial risk factors. Suggested questions for psychosocial screening are listed below. The groupings, namely 1–2, 3–5, 6–7, 8–9, and 10 correspond to depression, alcohol/substance abuse, domestic violence, parental history of abuse, and absence of social support, respectively (Costello *et al.*, 1988, Kemper & Kelleher, 1996).

SUGGESTED QUESTIONS FOR PSYCHOSOCIAL SCREENING

1. How often in the last week or two have you felt depressed?
2. In the past year, have you felt depressed for at least 2 weeks or more?

3. Have you had any problems with drinking over the last year?
4. Have you had any problems with drugs over the last year?
5. Have you tried to cut down on drinking or drugs?
6. Have you been emotionally or physically abused by your partner or someone important to you in the past year?
7. Have you been slapped, kicked, or otherwise physically hurt or are you afraid it might happen?
8. When you were a child, did your parents ever hurt you physically or emotionally?
9. Did your parents neglect you?
10. Do you have anyone you can count on to be dependable when you need help?

BIDIRECTIONAL INFLUENCES

Finally, the practitioner needs to consider the fact that the parent-child interaction is *bidirectional*, meaning that the child influences the family and environment, just as the family and environment influence the child. These influences can be risk-producing or protective in nature. This concept counters an issue frequently raised by parents in which they feel they have treated all their children the same, yet one child has a behavior problem, while the other does not. In actuality, they most likely *have not* treated both children the same. Birth order, addition of a new participant (i.e., sibling or siblings), change in household, or similar influences will also have an impact. Moreover, the child's own characteristic behaviors will alter how the parents respond to him or her (e.g., frequently irritable, slow to warm up, or being easily overstimulated). Development is multi-faceted; in addition to intrinsic or endogenous components found in the child, it is affected by maturation, learning, resolution of conflict (e.g., nurturance, security, autonomy), cognitive change, and adaptation to environmental demands.

Chapter 2

Parenting Issues

FAMILY CONSIDERATIONS

In the process of getting to know the child better, practitioners also need to learn more about the child's family. This is essential, in part because how parents deal with their child's behaviors will determine to a significant degree whether the behaviors lead to competent or incompetent social development in their children. Families are the most central and enduring influence in children's lives (Schor, 2002), and are a major source of stability and support for the child. They promote a sense of being "capable" in the child (Howard, 2002). This is accomplished via routines, providing models, instruction, progressive expectations, providing choices, role taking opportunities, and doling out appropriate consequences (Howard, 2002).

However, the family can also be a significant stressor. Being the "perfect parent" is an unattainable goal, and the quest for this idealized state often sets parents up for failure. Conversely, "bad parenting" is a label that is often unjustly bestowed on parents who are trying hard but who simply are ineffective. Parenting is a highly complex undertaking and there is no gold standard for success.

Parenting has its own developmental course that varies, depending on family composition. In a traditional, two-parent household, the first developmental stage involves becoming spouses and defining the parameters of relationships and interactions in the spouse subsystem. The birth of a child signals the advent of another role, namely, becoming the parent subsystem. The task facing the husband and wife is how to balance these two roles. Too much emphasis on the spouse role would leave the parents disengaged from the child and unwilling to meet the child's needs. On the other hand, sole emphasis on the parenting role would potentially stress the marital relationship and also prompt parents to reinforce excessive dependency by the child, as independence would diminish the need for the role to which the parents have dedicated themselves. Sole emphasis on the parenting role may also be a signal that the parents are avoiding intimacy that is inherent in the spouse role. The optimal situation occurs when parents successfully balance spouse and parent commitments.

The family constellation has changed dramatically over the last 40 years, with a five-fold increase in single parent households since 1960. More than one-third of children live in one-parent households at some point over the course of their lives, and this is higher in certain ethnic groups such as African-Americans. Divorce rates hover at approximately 50%, and the determining factor affecting children's adaptation to divorce is the quality of parenting that they continue to receive. Hence, the "typical" family of 30 years ago, namely, two parents and two children with the mother staying at home, is now a minority. As a result, single parents, blended families, other relatives being primary caretakers and divorce all have changed the complexion of the parenting unit and the developmental progression of the family. For example, with step-families, the husband and wife may never have had the opportunity to experience the spouse role prior to being thrust into being parents.

Schor (2002) has stated, "... the social tapestry supporting families has been weakened due to the considerable pressure and stress of the speed of social change." Parents have less time at home because of working longer and longer commutes, coupled with two-parent incomes. Interestingly, recent data indicate that parents spend the same amount of time with their children despite these pressures. This has to come at the cost of spousal relationships and time for oneself, raising the question as to whether time spent with the child is truly *quality* time. Parenting also involves provision of material support (food, clothing, shelter), instrumental support (safety, supervision, hygiene), social support (being cared for, loved, valued), socialization (guidance to connecting with the outside world), and education (coping skills, life skills) (Schor, 2002).

DIMENSIONS OF PARENTING

Overall parenting interactions can be separated into four basic dimensions (Baumrind, 1966, 1971, 1973) and it is important for both practitioners and parents to consider these when addressing behavioral concerns in the child. These dimensions are: (a) control, (b) communication, (c) maturity demands, and (d) nurturance.

Control

This parenting dimension refers to strictness of discipline, consistency, provision of clear directions, and limit setting. *Discipline* should be considered a process in which the child is taught what to do as well as what not to do, the ultimate goal being socialization. It includes a system of teaching, learning, and nurturing that encourages appropriate behavior and deters misbehavior. Essentially, parents should set limits and allow the child flexibility within those limits. When the parent gives a directive, the child has two choices: comply with the directive or protest/whine/ ignore it—in other words, be noncompliant. In such a situation, what the child does and how the parent responds is critical, because if the child does not comply and this lack of compliance is reinforced, then a more persistent behavioral pattern may evolve. Hence, discipline can be considered as a triangular configuration, the three components being reinforcement, consequences, and a positive parent-child relationship (Howard, 2002).

Control is on a continuum and ranges from extremely low to excessive. In the former, the parent might set a limit, but ultimately would give in if the child begged, whined, sweet-talked, or wheedled in a determined fashion. The child can therefore follow his own behavioral agenda. In the latter extreme, there simply is no tolerance for noncompliance. Parents should realize that provision of a reasonable degree of control is reluctantly welcomed by children, because it provides them with a stable base and a sense of security. It is analogous to the metaphor of a stoplight. While no one likes to wait at a red light, it is reassuring to know that things are predictable, and others will stop when they, in turn, get the red light. Without this consistency, drivers could stop or go regardless of the color of the stoplight making for a very unpredictable situation. Along these lines, a lack of limits also produces a state of unpredictability, and in fact often causes the child to test limits in new situations so as to gauge just how far to push issues.

Hoffman (1970) suggested that there are three types of control mechanisms. With *power assertion*, the parent uses threats, physical force, or withdrawal of privileges. The second mechanism is *love withdrawal* in which the parent will ignore, isolate, or refuse to speak to the child whose behaviors are "bad." This technique often incorporates the passive-aggressive, "silent treatment." Finally, there is the *induction* technique where the parent explains why the child's actions are "bad," using reasoning and emphasizing how the behavior would have a negative impact on others. Use of "if you keep screaming at your little brother, he will cry," is a good example of induction. Induction probably leads to the most prosocial behavior in children, although withdrawal of privileges arguably may need to accompany this technique in certain circumstances.

Several other issues are important when one considers the control dimension. First, children should be given choices, but the parent should pre-select the choice options. In the case of a simple parent-child interaction, it would be better for a parent to ask the child, "What would you like for breakfast, waffles or cereal?" versus simple asking, "What do you want for breakfast?" The former approach is proactive and would allow the child to feel as if she were in control, yet the control actually is external. With the latter, a battle might ensue if the child selects something that is not available or that the parent disagrees with.

In regard to problem behaviors, it would be appropriate for a parent to say, "If you don't stop crying you will have to leave the room" or "stop banging that toy on the floor or I'll have to take it away." This approach has the added benefit of teaching the child to make decisions and to develop a sense of responsibility for her actions. Invariably, a child will sometimes select the negative alternative so as to test the parent's control. Consistency is essential in such situations. Second, parents should have a sense of *parental presence*, namely, they should give the child the impression that they are in control. Constantly asking open-ended questions such as "can you stay in the waiting room while I speak to the doctor?" actually invites a negative response. Directives can be given in a firm, yet nurturing way such as "I'd like you to stay in the waiting room while I speak to the doctor." This is along the lines of a "declarative question," so to speak. Similarly, parental presence is not bolstered if the child is told, "you hurt mommy when you hit her." Although this does point out to the child that his behavior has an impact on others, this simply again places the child in control. In fact, at that moment, perhaps the child *did* want to impulsively strike out at the mother, and this simply reaffirms that she was successful. Using the third person technique such as, "when kids hit, they can hurt someone—and this is totally unacceptable," followed by a consequence, would be much more effective.

Finally, most misbehaviors are "low-key" aversive actions, and most parental responses are "low intensity" (e.g., a verbal warning). In fact, it is estimated that in toddlers and preschoolers, these low-key behaviors occur once every 4 to 8 minutes. This argues for the necessity of picking one's battles. If the parent consistently responds to the child's low-key behaviors with ineffective threats of consequences without follow-through, this behavioral pattern then becomes the child's modus operandi. More specifically, this pattern will be extrapolated to situations that are more significant, where the misbehaviors are more consequential. In other words, if parents try to control too many behaviors at once, they will be ineffective, inconsistent, and overwhelmed. Moreover, the likelihood of this ineffectiveness expanding to other situations is increased.

Communication

This dimension refers to the clarity of the parent-child communication. Communication reflects the parent's willingness to listen to a child's perspective as well as the parent giving reasons for actions and decisions. This dimension includes provision of reasons as to *why* the child should comply with the parent's directions. For example, it would be more effective for the parent to say, "go to bed because we all have to get up early tomorrow," than to simply state, "go to bed." Because communication is bi-directional, the parent should also listen (or at least acknowledge) the child's arguments as to why she should not have to go to bed. Parents who score low on the communication dimension typically would opt for the "because I said so" or "do as you're told" alternatives. There probably is a time for the "because I said so" option, this being restricted to situations where the child repeatedly tries to bargain or draw the parent into a debate or argument about a misbehavior and its consequence. This technique should be used after the child's point of view is acknowledged, but the line is drawn and the discussion is terminated.

Maturity Demands

This dimension reflects more of an implicit attitude in which parents expect the child to be responsible. Pressure, encouragement, achievement, and expectation to carry out duties are involved. Children are expected to do household tasks, homework, projects, and help parents when requested, without extrinsic rewards. In essence, the child is encouraged to be independent and to not act in ways that are deemed "babyish." Allowing the child to endure consequences of misbehavior (e.g., detention for not completing homework) is inherent in this dimension. Young children are encouraged to do things themselves, versus having the parents do it for them, if the behavior is reasonable and has a high likelihood of being completed by the child. Examples include getting dressed, washing hands, putting shoes on, or feeding a pet.

Nurturance

Nurturance involves warmth, control, and love. Reinforcement, support, and encouragement are components. Nurturance and communication are often intertwined, while to some parents, nurturance and control seem to be polarized opposites. More specifically, some parents see control as a withdrawal of nurturance and this mindset has to be addressed up-front by the practitioner. Conversely, it often is difficult for practitioners and parents to delineate when nurturance evolves into doting behavior. Fortunately, in most cases seen in our outpatient practice, parents have a higher tendency to be over- versus under-nurturing.

PARENTING PROFILES

Different combinations of these four dimensions of parenting have produced four primary parenting profiles (Baumrind, 1975, 1991, 1996).

Authoritarian Parenting

Authoritarian parents attempt to exert total control over their child's behaviors and attitudes. They are restrictive and demand conformity to absolute standards. Strict obedience, forceful punishment, strict rules, and intolerance of any challenge of authority are characteristics. These parents are high in the control and maturity demand dimensions, and low in nurturance and clarity of communication. These parents have a set standard of conduct that is extremely rigid, with rules being inflexible. Responsiveness to the child's needs is low, and the parents are highly directive. Obedience is valued as if it were a virtue, and "respect" is emphasized excessively. The authoritarian parent does not tolerate verbal give-and-take, believing the child should accept the parent's word in an unquestioning fashion. Power assertion and/or love withdrawal are often used in control maneuvers to gain compliance. These parents often are punitive and forceful. Their children often are classified as "conflicted-irritable," and are withdrawn, unable to make decisions, and unhappy with themselves and their social interactions. Some children of authoritarian parents may be passively hostile, sulky, unfriendly, and increasingly vulnerable to stress. They typically have lower self-esteem, poorer social skills, and increased levels of depression when compared to peers exposed to other parenting styles.

Permissive Parenting

Permissive parenting falls into two types: permissive-indulgent and permissive-indifferent. The *permissive-indulgent* parent places few demands or rules on the child; punishments are rare (or at best, inconsistent) and ineffectual. The parents do not act as role models, are non-controlling and non-demanding, yet they are warm and nurturant. They avoid confrontations, and allow the child to regulate her own behavior. Hence these parents are low on the control and maturity demand dimensions, and high in clarity of communication and nurturance. Parents offer no encouragement to obey family rules or external standards, and in doing so often back the child in conflicts with teachers, either implicitly or explicitly. The child is permitted to freely express her feelings and impulses without close monitoring. Communication is often taken to the extreme, that is, ad nauseum. Many parents are not aware that with young children in particular, after the first sentence or two of an explanation, the rest of the message is tuned out. Moreover, the explanation is sometimes misused as a disciplinary technique in and of itself, with the parent explaining why the child should not have engaged in a problem behavior, but not doing anything else about it. Children of permissive-indulgent parents are characterized as being "impulsive-aggressive" and typically are rebellious, have poor self control, are not self reliant, and often display poor academic achievement. They do not develop a sense of responsibility, in part because the parents often have bailed them out of situations in the past, so they were spared having to deal with consequences of their actions. These children often are perplexed about the fact that they are receiving poor grades, have not been picked for a team, or have to work to achieve a goal.

Permissive-indifferent parenting is characterized by a low degree of control and low maturity demands. The parents essentially are uninvolved with the child. Again, there are few rules, little structure, and minimal demands placed on the child. In contrast to the permissive-indulgent parent, parents who are permissive-indifferent also do not provide much nurturance, nor is there clarity of communication. Hence, all four dimensions of parenting are low. As a result, these parents appear more neglecting and more unresponsive, and this parenting style sometimes is referred to as "uninvolved parenting." The parenting style is lax and distant, and the family interactional style is classified as disengaged. Children from permissive-indifferent households often feel isolated and alienated, have poor self-control, and demonstrate a tendency to migrate toward undesirable peer groups. They tend to perform most poorly in all domains in comparison to peers raised under different parenting practices.

Authoritative Parenting

The *authoritative parenting* style is the most desirous. These parents direct their child's activities and behaviors rationally, and focus on issues, versus punishment. These parents are controlling, but explain their reasoning, and encourage verbal give-and-take with their child. The child's autonomous self-will and individuality are respected and valued, but firm control is exerted at the point of parent-child divergence. There are limits, but these are not overly restrictive. Standards and expectations are set for future conduct, and reason, as well as power, are employed to deal with potentially problematic behaviors. Hence, these parents are consistent, demanding, and firm. In essence, strong parental control is not incompatible with good socialization outcomes when high control and maturity demands are found in conjunction with high nurturance and clarity of communication. Authoritative parents also are willing to change their minds, if their decision was made in error, or if the child's viewpoint has merit. Children of these parents are considered "energetic-friendly" and are self-controlled, self-reliant, able to cope adequately with stress, cheerful and sociable, purposive, and achievement-oriented. They are classified as being *instrumentally competent.*

Stated differently, authoritarian parenting is more punitive and the focus is on gaining a child's obedience to parental demands, versus responding to the demands of the child (Baumrind, 1966, 1991). Permissive parents are more responsive to children, but do not set appropriate limits. Authoritative parents demonstrate a balanced approach that is more responsive to the child's needs, but still maintains a reasonable standard of conduct. The neglecting parent typically is uninvolved with the child and responds minimally to the child's needs or behaviors.

It therefore appears that authoritative parenting during the earlier years (e.g., preschool period) is associated with high cognitive and social competencies during school age in both males and females. Authoritarian parenting is associated with average cognitive and social competencies in school aged children of both sexes, while permissive parenting is related to low, subsequent cognitive and social competencies (with very low cognitive competencies in males) (Baumrind, 1975, 1991).

OTHER PARENTING ISSUES

Broadly defined, parenting refers to anything the parents do or fail to do that potentially affects their children. There is some debate regarding the distinction between *parenting style* and *parenting practice* (Brenner & Fox, 1999; Locke & Prinz, 2002). *Practice* refers to techniques or specific behaviors that have a direct effect on the development of behaviors in the child and which have a direct impact on the child's outcomes. *Style* is a constellation of attitudes toward the child that are communicated and create an emotional climate or context in which the parents' behaviors are expressed (Darling & Steinberg, 1993). Style is more indirect and is a moderator between practices and outcome (ultimate behaviors demonstrated by the child). Essentially, practice is *what* a parent does, while style is *how* they do it. Practices involve techniques such as time out, ignoring, or spanking. Style can be consistent-inconsistent, or strict-permissive.

Accordingly, Brenner and Fox (1999) report that parenting *practices* appear to aggregate into three clusters, based on parenting dimensions obtained from self-report measures such as the Parent Behavior Checklist (Fox, 1994). The three dimensions are discipline, nurturing practices, and expectations.

The first parenting cluster was characterized by high to very high discipline, low nurturing, and moderate to high expectations (Brenner & Fox, 1999). These parents punish frequently, expect more than their children are capable of doing, and spend little time engaged in nurturing behavior. This cluster resembles Baumrind's (1991) authoritarian parenting style. The second, most common cluster involved low to moderate scores on average amount of punishment doled out, moderate developmental expectations, and a moderate amount of time spent in nurturing activities. Interestingly, this cluster, found more with decreased education and lower socioeconomic status, has been considered "good-enough parenting" (Baumrind, 1991, 1996; Brenner & Fox, 1999). Children raised in either of these households typically had the most behavioral problems, and the parents employed verbal and corporal punishment (particularly in the first cluster). Fewer parents showed the third cluster, characterized by low to moderate discipline, high expectations, and high nurturing behavior (corresponding to the authoritative parenting style) or the fourth constellation of low discipline, high nurturing, and low expectations (permissive). It was also suggested that very high expectations could be positively expressed in encouragement of achievement, or, conversely, negatively result in excessive pressure to succeed that is overbearing to the child.

SUMMARY

First, practitioners and parents should realize that control is conducive to later social, emotional and intellectual competencies. However, as in the cases of authoritarian and authoritative parenting styles, *how* control is implemented or dispensed is a critical issue. In the former, it is presented in terms of domination; in the latter, it is firm but reasoned and flexible, if necessary. Laissez-faire parenting, seen in permissive profiles, is also problematic.

Stress

One must also consider that parenting styles are the result of bi-directional influences. For example, if the parent perceives that her child is lacking in coping skills or is easily overwhelmed by stress, then the parent may become more controlling, overprotective, and restrictive. Similarly, if the child is prone to explosiveness, parents may be less controlling in an effort to avoid conflicts. Both of these parental responses do not enhance positive developmental outcomes. In the former, preventing the child from experiencing stress or having an opportunity to learn to adjust to potentially stressful situations may be helpful in the short-term, but prevents him from developing social and adaptive skills that will be needed in the future. As mentioned previously, a mild degree of stress enhances problem-solving and serves as an "inoculation" of sorts, enhancing development of stress-fighting "antibodies" that can also be employed in the future. With respect to the latter avoidance of conflict response, the child will not learn limit setting under the protective auspices of the family, and will simply generalize this maladaptive response pattern and apply it to other situations. In the former case where the child is perceived to lack coping skills, control/restrictiveness will need to gradually be decreased. In the latter more explosive situation, control/restrictiveness will need to be increased.

Both parents need to be on the same page with respect to parenting styles, this being termed "inter-agent consistency." If the mother is high with respect to control, but the father is low, this might cause polarization in terms of this dimension of parenting. The mother would see the father as being too lenient, thereby becoming even more controlling. The father, on the other hand, very well might respond to this increased control by being even more permissive, thereby promulgating a recurrent cycle of maladaptive, conflictual parenting behavior. Clinical experience has shown that discrepancies in preferred parenting techniques sometimes provide the means by which parents address conflicts between themselves, namely, it could be a way to passively or indirectly anger the other parent. Such "detouring" of conflict must be a consideration whenever the practitioner evaluates parenting profiles.

Using a family stress model, stress from the environment (e.g., job-related, financial, housing) can have two pathways leading to: (1) parental emotional distress, or (2) marital conflict or instability. Either of these courses will, in turn, lead to disrupted parenting, the end result being poor child emotional and behavioral outcomes.

Parental History

The parents' own histories also often influence their current parenting styles, however this varies on a case-by-case basis. Some parents who have been subject to authoritarian parenting when they, themselves, were younger often employ similar parenting techniques; conversely, a significant number of these individuals comprehend the negative impact of such child rearing practices and opt for the other extreme, namely, they become more permissive. Clinically, it is highly infrequent to encounter a case in which the parent has been raised in a permissive household but then embraces an authoritarian parenting style with her own children. Parents frequently engage in behavioral patterns with their children that trigger a re-experiencing of a conflict or stress that was encountered earlier in their own childhood. This type of pattern is usually unacknowledged (i.e., unconscious), emotionally charged, negative, and it occurs repeatedly. For example, if a parent were raised in a punitive, overly controlling family, strivings for independence in his own child would be troubling. Parents' own aspirations, unachieved goals, or current areas of day-to-day stress all may influence their *excessive* emphasis on the child participating in sports, sociability issues, or academic achievement.

For example, in a 6-year study where parent psychological problems were broadly defined, if both the mother and father were negative for a psychologic diagnosis, 36% of the offspring had a behavioral or psychologic problem; if the mother was negative for a psychologic problem, but the father was positive, there was a 47% prevalence rate in the child. However, if the mother was positive and the father negative for psychologic difficulties, the rate of problems in their children was 68%, and if both parents were positive, it was 72% (Schor, 2002).

Other Parental Risks

Another common pitfall in parenting that may negatively affect the parent-child relationship involves attributing adult-like motives and thinking to the child. Statements such as "she's crying to make me angry" or "he's doing that to be mean," which are proffered as explanations of the behavior of an infant or young child are clues of parental misperceptions that need to be addressed immediately by the practitioner. Related to this is the situation when a parent inappropriately takes to heart statements from a toddler such as "I hate you" or "You should go away," these typically said when the toddler was angry. Informing the parent that the child doesn't understand the true meaning or impact of the words he is saying and that the child has learned that such statements get a response (even though the child is clueless as to what the statements mean) would be extremely helpful.

Parents should also adjust parenting behaviors directed toward the child, based on the child's developmental maturity level. In general, there is a shift from routine caretaking (physical needs) to non-caretaking activities (reasoning, discussion) that occurs in a gradual fashion. A lack of rules, failure to monitor the child, use of erratic punishment, and reward compromise are components of a particular cluster of parenting behaviors that lead to conduct problems.

Therefore, when considering "minimal competency" in parenting, several risk factors emerge from a review of the literature (e.g., Budd & Holdsworth, 1996). While the presence of these risk factors does not necessarily indicate incompetent parenting, the *possibility* of such increases directly in proportion to the number of these risk factors that are present. These parenting risk factors that practitioners should evaluate in a detailed history are:

- negative past events (history of being abused, violence in adult relationships, previous incidents of abusive behavior directed toward a child)
- greater number of abusive caregivers a parent had during childhood
- limited intellectual functioning of parent (this is more likely to be related to subsequent neglect than abuse)
- presence of emotional disorders/personality disorders
- chronic unemployment, few/poor social relationships and supports (particularly in conjunction with high family stress)
- naivete about child development, unrealistic expectations of children stress/unhappiness about the parenting role
- conflicted marriage
- coercive and controlling interactions
- poor parental response to previous intervention (if applicable)
- alcoholism/drug use
- poverty
- limited privacy/insufficient personal time
- responsibilities for extended family members
- job stresses/dissatisfaction

Practitioners should also assess parenting strengths such as interpersonal skills, affective involvement with the child, supportive extended family relationships, and the parent's sincere desire to improve parenting skills (Budd & Holdsworth, 1996).

Discipline

Parents must also distinguish *discipline* from *punishment*, as this distinction is critical in terms of how a child's behaviors are dealt with. As suggested earlier, it should be underscored that discipline be thought of as the framework or structure that the caretaker puts in place, designed to enable the child to fit into the real world in a positive and effective manner. The purpose of discipline (caretaking behavior) is to teach a child what *to* do and what *not* to do. Discipline involves methods to discourage inappropriate behavior and to foster appropriate behavior. Some disciplinary techniques are more effective than others, with ineffective methods sometimes actually becoming reinforcing to the child for his misbehavior. Ineffective discipline is sometimes deemed dysfunctional, maladaptive, or inept (Kendziora & O'Leary, 1993; Patterson, 1986). Stated differently, discipline teaches a child how to behave, so as to enhance socialization. It is instruction that is instilled in the child, versus rigidly imposed on him, the goal being to have the child subsequently develop his or her own self-discipline. Because children below the age of 4–5 years of age generally have not internalized self-discipline, use of external discipline is particularly critical at this time. In other words, discipline instilled by parents is the foundation for the child's self discipline later. Punishment may be a component of discipline, the purpose being to reduce misbehavior; however, it is not the main component. Discipline can consist of more desirable positive approaches such as use of praise, reasoning, compromising, and teaching, or it can be more negative and involve less desirable techniques such as yelling, spanking, shaming, or ridiculing.

Discipline and nurturance are two of the most heavily investigated constructs in parenting research (Locke & Prinz, 2002). Ineffective discipline is implicated in conduct disorders and delinquency, poor academic achievement, substance abuse and related problems; nurturance is related to the more positive dimensions of secure attachment, school readiness, good academic performance, and prosocial development. Nurturance in parenting provides a positive atmosphere for the parent-child relationship and the child's emotional development. It can be demonstrated by emotional experiences (hugs, verbal statements of love and support, communication of acceptance) or by instrumental acts (special time, playing a game together) (Locke & Prinz, 2002).

Finally, the unstated goal of parenting is to develop so-called *instrumental competence* in the child (Baumrind, 1973). This is defined as social responsibility, friendliness, independence, achievement-orientation, vitality, being energetic, and displaying empathic, prosocial activities. The impact of parenting has long-term ramifications with regard to cognitive competency (taking on challenges, being motivated to achieve), as well as social skills. The end result is to have the child become a well-adjusted individual who is able to successfully maneuver in the outside world.

Chapter 3

Child Characteristics

The course of development depends on the synthesis of the influences of intrinsic/endogenous factors and environment/learning (Aylward, 1992b). The former includes genetic endowment, IQ, physical characteristics, and temperament. The latter involves sociocultural aspects, family interactions, parenting, and peer influences. How these influences meld will determine cognitive, personality and social development in the young child. This combination will also determine the development of behavioral problems.

Generally, the first $1\frac{1}{2}$ to 2 years is considered to be the infancy period. The toddler stage ranges from approximately 18 months to age 3-years, and early childhood spans the three up to 6-year age range. Development during these stages is a process of qualitative change, whereby the child initially depends on caretakers and the environment for nurturance, security, and attachment. A subsequent separation from caretakers and establishment of autonomy and a sense of mastery occur, followed by heightened interest in peer and social interactions. Motor and cognitive functioning diverge, and language assumes an increasingly important role (Aylward, 1997). Many developmental acquisitions occur over this time span. Some, such as ambulation, language acquisition, and toilet training, are obvious; others including development of object permanency, causality, imitation, and symbolic thinking are more subtle. Many problem behaviors that cause parental concern may be age-related normal behaviors that involve the aforementioned issues. They may also be reactions to family stresses.

COGNITIVE ABILITIES

The child's stage of cognitive, social and emotional development has a major impact on overt behaviors. Cognitive development progresses from the sensorimotor stage (first 18–24 months) to the preoperational stage (2–6 years), to the stage of concrete operations (6–11 years)

(Piaget & Inhelder, 1969). Each stage is characterized by distinct cognitive processes or ways of thinking. Characteristics of the sensorimotor stage include development of imitation, language, object permanency, fine motor/visual motor skills, goal-directed behaviors, and problem solving. Two processes enable the child to adapt to environmental demands: *assimilation* and *accommodation*. Assimilation involves matching new information to already existing cognitive structures, while accommodation involves altering cognitive structures to take in new information. Play is considered to be pure assimilation, while imitation is pure accommodation. The interplay between these two constructs determines how a child thinks and learns in new situations.

For example, if information is too complex for a child to understand, he or she will interpret it at a more developmentally immature level (assimilation). That is why long-winded parental explanations often are misunderstood and why parents and professionals must be careful in how they frame information for the child (including descriptions of illness). However, if the information is just slightly above the child's present cognitive level, he may develop new understandings or cognitive "structures" (schemas) in response, via the process of accommodation. For example, a very young child may have the cognitive schema that anything that flies is a bird. When she first sees a butterfly, she might assimilate that information and also call the insect a bird. After correction by the mother and perhaps additional sightings of both birds and butterflies, the child will accommodate and develop a new schema that brightly colored, smaller creatures that float, versus fly, are indeed butterflies.

In the preoperational period, qualitative differences in thinking between the adult and child become apparent. *Egocentricity* is the inability to take another's point of view, and this can explain why a child might want to buy a matchbox car for his father on Christmas (why not—*I'd* like it), or the fact that the child might think she caused her parents' divorce, or was responsible for an illness or hospitalization. *Realism* refers to the child's inability to separate thoughts from reality (sometimes making it difficult to differentiate this confusion from lying; this also causes difficulty for children to recount a traumatic incident accurately after several interviews). *Animism* infers that anything that moves is alive (explaining some fears), and *centration* makes it difficult for a child to understand that he lives in a town that is part of a state, which in turn is part of the United States (or that daddy is grandpa's son). Children are affected by *states versus transformations*, and perceptions override reasoning. As a result, "transformer" toys are fascinating because after a few manipulations, they assume different end states. Similarly, even though the child might initially put on a Halloween mask, when she sees herself in the mirror, the mask (not the child underneath it) is the predominant impression, typically causing the child to wear the costume *without* a mask. Words are interpreted literally, thus making the child particularly vulnerable to a derogatory comment made by a peer, parent, or teacher (such as calling him "stupid"). This would also explain the child being fascinated by riddles, or confused by terms such as "headlight" or "Miami" (your "ami"?). There is no understanding of time concepts (e.g., we'll go in a few hours), or death. The ability to abstract is not apparent even in the concrete operational period (ages 7–11). It is not until a *mental age* of 11 that a child can abstract, develop hypotheses, and deal with concepts such as transitivity (A = B, B = C, therefore A = C), this being the formal operational period. Obviously, the child's cognitive abilities will have an impact on behavioral issues as well.

TEMPERAMENT

Temperament is defined as the child's behavioral style or the "how" of behavior (Thomas & Chess, 1980); it does not address the "why" (motivations) or "what" (abilities or developmental level). Temperament involves the way a child behaves, both spontaneously and in reaction to the environment or situations, and is best conceptualized as an organizing principle in children's physiologic responses to environmental challenges. The infant is born with a specific temperament, and it is likely that the components of temperament are derived from genetic factors that interact with the environment and the child's physical state. Although these traits are relatively stable, they are not entirely fixed, again underscoring the bi-directional nature of caretaker-infant interaction. Measurement of temperament can be accomplished by parental interview, questionnaires (Carey & McDevitt, 1995a; Medloff-Cooper, Carey, & McDevitt, 1995), and the clinician's own behavioral observations (Aylward, 1992a; Carey & McDevitt, 1995b).

The interest in temperament was derived from the 1956 New York Longitudinal Study (NYLS) (Thomas & Chess, 1980). From infant behavioral records obtained in the NYLS, nine categories of temperament were established (Chess & Thomas, 1996, 1999). These are:

- *Activity level:* Motor component; diurnal proportion of active and inactive periods (motility during eating, playing, bathing, sleep-wake cycle, ambulation). Too high of an activity level would potentially be problematic.
- *Rhythmicity (regularity):* Predictability/unpredictability of functions (hunger, feeding pattern, elimination, sleep-wake cycle).

Infants with low rhythmicity would have good and bad days without any pattern or predictability.

- *Approach/withdrawal:* Characteristic nature of the initial response to a new stimulus (e.g., food or toy) or person. This could be positive (approach) or negative (withdrawal), with the latter being less desirable.
- *Adaptability:* Responses to new or different situations (ease in which initial response can be positively modified). This category involves the child's tolerance to change and difficulty with transitions, with poor adaptability being viewed negatively.
- *Threshold of responsiveness:* Intensity level of stimulation needed to elicit a response, or sensitivity (reactions to sensory stimuli, environmental objects, social interaction). Low threshold causes overstimulation, perhaps related to sensory integration issues.
- *Intensity of reaction:* Response energy level (positive or negative). Forceful, loud not viewed positively.
- *Quality of mood:* Positive (friendly, happy) versus negative (unfriendly, crying).
- *Distractibility:* Degree to which extraneous environmental stimuli interfere with goal-directed behavior. Inability to focus behavior and attention.
- *Attention span/persistence:* Length of time an activity is pursued by child and continuation with that activity when faced with obstacles ("singlemindedness," ability to "stick-to-it"). Negative would be whining, nagging, locked-in behaviors that often are termed stubborn.

Interestingly, these same categorizations have been employed with the NYLS subjects in adolescence and early adulthood. From these nine temperament categories, three functional constellations of temperament have been identified (Chess & Thomas, 1999). These constellations are described below.

Temperament Constellations

Easy Child

The *easy child* constellation, found in approximately 40% of the population, is characterized by regularity, positive approach responses to new stimuli, high adaptability to change, and a predominantly positive mood (of mild to moderate intensity). These children adapt smoothly and without tension to parental standards, and generally have few behavioral problems. They are predictable with regard to sleep, eating, and elimination schedules, and readily adjust to new situations and people. When children with an easy child temperamental style do develop behavioral problems, the clinician must consider situational stresses.

Difficult Child

At the opposite end of the continuum is the *difficult child* constellation, which comprises approximately 10% of the population. Characteristics include irregularity in biological functions, negative withdrawal responses to new stimuli or people, poor adaptability to change, and primarily negative mood expressions that are intense (although even laughing is loud and excessive). These children typically demonstrate unpredictable hunger and sleep patterns, non-acceptance of new foods, prolonged periods necessary for adjustment, and frequent, loud crying. Children with a difficult child temperamental style are prone to temper tantrums, do not adjust well to changes in routines, and are easily frustrated.

While this temperamental constellation is not pathologic per se, a child manifesting this temperamental style is most vulnerable to behavioral problems in early and middle childhood, with 70% having clinically evident behavior disorders before 10 years of age (usually of a mild to moderate severity). Parental attitudes and practices that are effective with most children are not useful here, and inconsistency, loss of patience, punitiveness, or permissiveness often result. Parents may feel inadequate in their parenting role and thus be threatened and anxious, they may blame the infant or child and resent the burdens placed on the family, or they may simply be intimidated, and therefore routinely give in to the child's demands so as to avoid confrontation. Oppositional-defiant disorders, colic, and attention deficit hyperactivity disorders are associated with this temperamental style. A child with a difficult temperament who also has mental retardation, a language disorder, physical handicap, or a chronic medical condition would be even more demanding on parents and also at heightened risk for behavioral problems.

Slow-to-Warm-Up Child

Slow-to-warm-up children comprise approximately 15% of the population, and display negative responses of a mild intensity to new stimuli, slow but eventual adaptability, and a tendency toward irregularity of biologic function. If given the opportunity to re-experience situations in a gradual manner, these children eventually are more accepting.

Conversely, if pressured by parental insistence on an immediate positive response to a new food, place, or person, the child will become
stressed and will withdraw. Obviously, this can evolve into a vicious
cycle. Clinically, these children often demand more transition objects
(e.g., "blankies," pacifiers, stuffed animals). Teachers may underestimate
abilities of these children because of their reluctance to participate in
classroom activities, and they often experience difficulty in adjusting to
preschool or kindergarten.

    As is readily apparent, 35% of children do not fit any of these three
constellations of temperament, but nonetheless may display a preponder-
ance of behaviors that resemble, but do not totally fit, the three categorizations. The temperamental constellations represent behavioral
variations that are within normal limits, and which underscore the wide
range of "normal."

Temperament and Problem Behaviors

With respect to how temperament might contribute to problem behaviors,
one must consider a goodness-of-fit conceptualization (Chess & Thomas,
1999). Goodness-of-fit involves a matching of environmental properties
(expectations, demands) with the child's capacities and behavioral predispositions. *Consonance* exists when a match occurs between the environment and child's reactivity; *dissonance* appears when there is a mismatch
among the two. So-called poorness-of-fit between the environment and
the child's temperament results in excessive stress, and behavioral disorders are thought to be the result of such a mismatch between temperament,
capacities, and environment. For example, if parents are more low-key
and retiring, and the child is overly active, and displays characteristics of
a difficult child temperamental style, then dissonance results; conversely,
if the parents are more of a so-called "type-A" personality, and the child
manifests a slow-to-warm-up temperamental style, a mismatch again
occurs. This underscores the concept of bi-directional influences and the
fact that no single set of child behavior management techniques is optimal
for all children.

    Consideration of temperament allows the practitioner and parents
to view the child from a clearer perspective (Carey, 1982). Emphasis is
placed on normality, versus abnormality, the child's behaviors are better
understood, and blame is avoided. Rather than have the parents blame
themselves for purported "bad parenting," emphasis on the inborn nature
of behavioral predispositions can be reassuring. Such an approach also
is helpful in delineating the child's contribution to behavior problems,

and provides an entrée into anticipatory guidance. The clinician could also consider temperament when providing advice on weaning and toilet training, evaluating a child's reaction to illness, and discussing behavioral concerns that simply might fall between a normal developmental variation and a problem (e.g., hyperactivity, sleep difficulties, negativism). How a child adjusts to nursery school or kindergarten, establishes peer relations, and approaches academics, all can be framed in the context of temperament. It is easy to see how low sensory thresholds, a tendency toward withdrawal, or high intensity of reaction could contribute to behavioral problems, even during infancy.

Excellent management approaches in dealing with the child's temperamental qualities and temperamental styles have been delineated by Chess and Thomas (1996, 1999), Carey and Jablow (1997), and Turecki and Tonner (1989). For example, with the easy child, parents need to monitor minor complaints that are related to physical issues, social interactions, or academic activities. Because these children are not prone to vigorous protests and adjust to even moderate discomfort, problems are not brought to the parents' attention and therefore are easily overlooked. With regard to the slow-to-warm-up child, she should be provided with familiarity of a situation before being thrust into it (e.g., visiting a new school and meeting the teacher prior to the first day of school). Avoidance of hurrying the child is highly important, as is identification of as many situations as possible in which the child's self esteem and self-confidence can be strengthened. Parents of a child with a difficult temperament should anticipate the child's withdrawing and negative tendencies, and should take care not to accelerate tantrums into chaos by reacting excessively themselves. On the other hand, they should maintain structure and impose discipline, rather than give in to the child's demands. It sometimes is difficult to differentiate legitimate complaints from whining or negative mood, requiring parents to carefully monitor the child's behaviors.

Other Temperamental Considerations

Studies seeking to further understand the contributions of biological and genetic factors to temperament involve salivary cortisol (Gunnar, 1990, 1994), vagal tone (Porges, 1992), EEG activation, and twin studies such as the MacArthur Longitudinal Twin Study. It is estimated that genetics accounts for 30%–40% of the differences in temperament, and 20%–30% of individual differences in emotional characteristics.

It appears that the most stable temperamental characteristics involve approach/withdrawal, mood, and activity and these characteristics appear to be under genetic control (Kagan, 1992; Kagan & Snidman, 1991). The former is assumed to reflect differential thresholds in the limbic system to novel and challenging events (Kagan et al., 1988). More specifically, the amygdala and its projections to the corpus striatum, hypothalamus, cingulated cortex, central gray and sympathetic nervous system are involved (Kagan, 1992). Moreover, early demonstration of frequent crying accompanied by high motor activity at 4-months of age is related to high levels of fear in later infancy. Different temperaments have also been related to different EEG measurements in the left and right anterior areas of the brain, although it is not clear whether EEG drives behavior, or vice versa. Increased right frontal activity (in comparison to the left) has been associated with increased distress in response to mild stress, and less happiness in infants.

ATTACHMENT

The complex "dance" between infant characteristics (temperament) and parenting is demonstrated in *attachment*. Attachment was first emphasized by Bowlby (1969), and underscores the importance of early relationships on the child's social and emotional development. Attachment is best described as the enduring affective bond that develops over time between the child and caregivers. Early on it is biologically based and involves sucking, crying, smiling, clinging and visual and locomotor following. These behaviors activate maternal responsive behavior, which then reciprocally increases attachment behaviors on the part of the child. The reactivity of the infant to the caretaker, its physical appearance, and the degree of demand the infant places on the caretaker will, in addition to the caretaker's own attributes, affect attachment. Simply stated, a "rewarding" infant will increase the possibility of a strong attachment over time; conversely, an infant whose behavior is non-rewarding to the caretaker would decrease this possibility. Therefore, although attachment is developed by means of child characteristics and interactions, the behavior that results can be thought of as a characteristic of the child. Rutter (1995) has demonstrated the clinical validity of attachment.

Parent-child synchrony (reciprocal social interactions) can easily be disrupted by temperamental styles in a bi-directional manner. The transactional approach (Sameroff & Chandler, 1978) accounts for variability in the attachment process, which varies as a function of the infant's behavior and caretaker responses to the behavior. While there are normal developmental sequences to attachment, the landmark work of Ainsworth (Ainsworth, 1979; Ainsworth, Blehar, Waters, & Wall, 1978) has been most useful for the practitioner. By means of Ainsworth's experimental work, three basic types of attachment have been identified, and behavioral indicators of these types are often evident in informal clinical observation.

Secure Attachment

In *secure attachment* the infant uses the mother as a secure base from which to explore the environment. The child may initially be wary of strangers, tends to become upset and protest if the mother leaves, and calms quickly and is very happy upon her return. On the caretaker side, mothers of these infants deal promptly and appropriately with their baby's needs, with the mother being "tuned in" to her infant.

Insecure Attachment

Insecurely attached babies fall into two groups: *insecure-ambivalent* and *insecure-avoidant*. In the former group, infants sometimes approach and cling to the mother, yet at other times push away. They may ask for help but then become angry when it is offered. These babies often resist their parents' attempts to console them and parents typically are unable to fully comfort them. On separation, the child's reaction to being reunited with the mother varies, with aggression occasionally being evident. These infants may either appear angrier than their peers or they may be conspicuously passive. Mothers of insecure-ambivalent children typically are inconsistent in their responses: at times they ignore the infant's cues, whereas on other occasions, they are responsive to the infant's signals. Responsivity depends on the mother's needs and mood at any given time. Insecure-avoidant children often fail to seek proximity with their caretaker and display very independent behavior. They do not cry when separated from the mother and when reunited, frequently ignore the mother altogether. They treat strangers much as they treat the mother, perhaps with less avoidance. On some occasions they react to the mother with gaze aversion or distancing. These mothers are highly insensitive to the baby's signals and avoid close contact with the child, rarely showing affection or emotional expression. Neglected and maltreated infants often develop insecure attachments.

Disorganized Attachment

Another attachment status, *disorganized attachment*, has been identified. These babies demonstrate more disorganized, often bizarre, conflict behaviors directed toward caretakers, especially under stress. These infants also may have one of the other insecure attachment patterns as the primary underlying pattern. In general, attachment patterns are relationship-specific versus trait-like, meaning that the infant can have different attachments to different primary caregivers (Steele, Steele, & Fonagy, 1996). In addition, attachments can change over time, with some ambivalent infants becoming avoidant as they get older. However, if the caretaker-child interaction improves, so can the degree of attachment, and this has been seen in children from orphanages who were adopted at age 4 years and still developed secure attachments with their caretakers. Moreover, securely attached infants adjust better cognitively and socially than do their insecurely attached counterparts. They cooperate better with caretakers, are more willing to learn new skills and try new activities, comply with rules, and seek help from parents. They are better able to adapt to school at age 5 years. Insecure-ambivalent children may not learn well from their parents and respond with anger and resistance to their parents' attempts to help or teach them. They often invest so much energy in conflicts that there is little left for other pursuits. Children with insecure-avoidant attachment tend to simply passively tune-out parents. In general, less securely attached children do not adjust well to preschool, some being very dependent, while others chronically complain and whine. While the relationship between temperament and attachment is not clear, in addition to infant temperamental style, maternal characteristics of self-centeredness, adaptability, persistence, perception of effectiveness, physical health and emotional state, are influential.

In summary, practitioners should also consider problematic attachment as a possible etiologic factor in the development of behavioral problems. This is especially true in children under 5-years of age, because early relationships are critical modulators of behavior in these children (Boris, Fueyo, & Zeanah, 1997; Cassidy, 1994).

CLINICAL EVALUATION OF ATTACHMENT

Boris et al. (1997) and Zeanah et al. (1993) provide excellent suggestions for the clinical evaluation of attachment in the office setting. First, the child's style of showing affection and seeking comfort from the parent should be monitored. Concern is raised if the child: (1) demonstrates a lack of affectionate interchanges with the parent, (2) displays indiscriminant affect toward strangers, or (3) demonstrates the pattern of not seeking comfort when distressed or showing increased distress while simultaneously seeking close proximity to the caregiver (ambivalent reaction) (Boris et al., 1997).

Second, Boris et al. (1997) emphasize the importance of how the child relies on the caregiver for help and the degree of cooperation between parent and child. Either excessive dependence on the caregiver, or the inability to pursue and employ the supportive presence of the parent to whom the child is attached is a cause for concern.

Exploratory behavior, in terms of the child checking back with the parent (physically with younger children; visually referencing with older children) or excessive unwillingness to leave the caregiver should be monitored. So-called *reunion responses* are particularly important, with avoidance, angry resistance, fearfulness, or lack of affection being indicative of major problems.

The child's history should be reviewed for the presence of the following risks to adequate attachment: (1) prolonged separations from parents during the first 3 years; (2) any abuse or neglect; or (3) membership in the following risk groups: those with a history of failure to thrive, sleep disorders, prenatal drug exposure, or having a depressed mother (particularly during infancy or the preschool period) (Boris et al., 1997).

Practitioners should observe the parents' actual and stated approach to the child, the caretaker-child interaction, how the parent describes the child and the child's behaviors, and the young patient's reaction to the clinician. This can be accomplished with incidental observations in the waiting area or examination room.

VULNERABLE CHILD SYNDROME

The *vulnerable child syndrome* (Green, 1986; Green & Solnit, 1964) was first identified almost 40 years ago, and is characterized by difficulty with separation, overprotectiveness, bodily overconcerns, and later school underachievement. Children at risk for this syndrome are those: (a) who had experienced a life-threatening illness (e.g., prematurity, accident, hospitalization, where the parent feared the child might die); (b) who represented for the parent a significant person from the past who died (e.g., sibling, parent's sibling); (c) whose life or mother's life was at risk during pregnancy and delivery (e.g., abruptio placenta, mother informed during pregnancy that the fetus might die in utero); or (d) those children whose mothers have a history of difficult pregnancies (miscarriages, stillbirths). At particular risk are older parents with many years of infertility, or young, single mothers without support of relatives.

Other indicators associated with this syndrome include rare use of babysitters (often restricted only to relatives), significant limitations or restrictiveness placed on the child's activities, parents' inability to set age-appropriate limits, and sleep problems (child sleeps in the parents' bed, parent awakens several times per night to check on the child). Parents of vulnerable children are overprotective, overindulgent, over-vigilant and over-solicitous. They experience separation anxiety, perceive the child as being younger that she/he actually is, and often forbid participation in bicycling or sports for fear of potential injury. The child is thought to be "sickly," and there is inordinate worry regarding "paleness," "blueness," fatigability, or circles under the child's eyes. Out-of-control behavior is often seen only in the parent(s)' presence, and this includes argumenta-tiveness and physical aggressiveness by the child that is directed toward the parent. Here the parent loses the aforementioned *parental presence*, or the nonverbal projection of an effective, "in control" mother or father. Complaints of hyperactivity are often raised and other children in the fam-ily often are not affected. Other potential clues as to the presence of this syndrome include parents whose reasons for visits to the physician are unclear, and those whose concerns for the child are frequently greater than what is actually warranted. As a result, there is overuse of medical serv-ices, doctor shopping, and anticipatory grief is rekindled when the child is ill. The child becomes cognizant that the parents are fearful, even though the parents' expectation of vulnerability might be subtle. The inhibitory reservations essentially limit the child's independence and autonomy, frequently resulting in later school refusal and learning difficulties.

Oftentimes, the relationship between the child's symptoms and past issues are not obvious (Green, 1986). Asking if the child was ever seriously ill, what the doctor told the parents about the child's condition, and if the parents feared the child might die provides useful information. Using third-person explanations and examples is also helpful in manage-ment. Prevention of the initiation of a vulnerable child classification is preferable and effective. This can be accomplished by judicious use of diagnostic evaluations, exquisite explanation of test results, and provi-sion of a clear, unequivocal summary of the child's current health status and vulnerability to potential problems in the future (Leslie & Boyce, 1996).

There are several variants of the vulnerable child syndrome which dif-fer only in the fact that the parent believes that a child is unusually suscep-tible to illness but not be especially worried about the child actually dying (Green, 1986). These variants include: (a) the illness prone child (as much as 40% do not have any illness); (b) pseudo-fever of unknown origin (tem-peratures in the normal range misjudged to be a low-grade fever, due in part to excessively frequent temperature-taking); (c) non-disease (e.g., innocent murmur that is interpreted by parents as heart disease); (d) familial sus-ceptibility (serious illness has previously occurred in the child or another family member); or (e) chronic illness of a non-life threatening nature.

Parental perception of child vulnerability (PPCV) (Thomasgard & Metz, 1995) may be heightened because of certain early health events such as pregnancy, prematurity, congenital heart disease, false positive test results (e.g., PKU) and jaundice. This is expanded during the first 5-years of life to include colic, feeding and crying problems, self-limited infectious illnesses (e.g., croup) and hospitalization. Marital dissatisfaction could also exacerbate PPCV. As a result, clinicians may want to consider use of the 8-item Child Vulnerability Scale (Forsyth, Leaf, Horwitz, & Leventhal, 1993), or the 16-item Vulnerable Child Scale (Perrin, West, & Cully, 1989).

SPOILED CHILD SYNDROME

Practitioners will frequently hear the term, "spoiled," despite the fact that there is no clearly defined meaning (in part because the term is negative and derogatory). However, the *spoiled child syndrome* (McIntosh, 1989) can be operationally defined and is characterized by excessive, self-centered and immature behavior. It includes a lack of consideration for others, demands to have one's own way, proneness to temper outbursts, and difficulty in delaying gratification. Behaviors are considered obstructive, intrusive, and manipulative, and these children are not easily satisfied and generally are unpleasant to be around. It is postulated that this syndrome is the result of parents not enforcing consistent, age-appropriate limits, however, it is quite likely that temperament also contributes. The degree of so-called spoiling varies from mild to severe and the type of problem behavior depends on the child's developmental stage. Early indicators of mild spoiling include trained night feeding (after 4–5 months of age) and trained night crying (older than 4 months). Recurrent temper tantrums may also be a sign of spoiling; *recurrent* is the key word, as most children will display a temper tantrum at one time or another. The most extreme case of the spoiled child syndrome is the child who is out of control. In this situation, the infant throws frequent temper tantrums, is physically aggressive, destructive, and oppositional/defiant. Refusal to comply with simple demands of daily living is common. This problem can be viewed on a continuum ranging from mild to severe, with the severe form of spoiling resembling an oppositional-defiant disorder.

SUMMARY

Child-Caretaker Interplay

It becomes apparent that the child has inborn characteristics that will influence caretaker reactions. Conversely, caretakers' reactions will, to some extent, determine whether the child's behavioral characteristics are maintained, become attenuated, or intensify. Superimposed on this interplay are normal, age-specific developmental issues. Using Erikson's (1963) theory, each stage of development represents a so-called critical period of conflict between positive and negative developmental possibilities. How the child balances the demands of the environment and his own developmental drives at each stage will set the course for future stages of development. Development of trust and a sense of security early on will form the basis for later development of autonomy. Autonomy, in turn, will provide the basis for the child to develop initiative, and so on. (See Chapter 5.) Besides how the environmental reacts to the infant or child, his or her own characteristics will drive how each developmental issue is handled and resolved. For example, temperament will affect how a child exerts autonomy; while attachment modulates the development of trust. Cognitive skills will affect the child's drive for mastery over a situation. Without doubt, the various profiles or configurations of these influences help to explain the wide range of normality and uniqueness found in children.

Characteristics of Invulnerability

Finally, some children do well, despite adverse circumstances, this being labeled as *invulnerability* or *resilience*. Characteristics of these children include:

- Internal locus of control (perception by the child that he has some control or impact on what happens in his life)
- Positive self-esteem
- Achievement-oriented
- Sense of responsibility
- Social maturity
- Outside interests
- Sense of humor
- Flexible coping strategies

It is good practice to foster development of these behaviors in all children, as they will have a major, positive impact on overall development.

Chapter 4

Externalizing Disorders

When the child's behaviors become problematic and affect family, social, and educational functions, they often are referred to as *Disruptive Behavior Disorders* (DBD) or *Externalizing Disorders*. In many respects, disruptive or externalizing disorders reflect the prototypal scenario of how the combination of: (a) problematic infant/child characteristics and behaviors, with (b) maladaptive parenting responses and contributions, results in significant problems. Disruptive, externalizing disorders are the single, most common cause of referral for mental health services. Moreover, these behaviors are among the most stable and therefore portend the possibility of heightened risk for later problems. For example, if a child demonstrates disruptive, aggressive behavior at age 7, there is a 50% risk that these behaviors will be present during adolescence. Stated differently, it is rare to find an antisocial adult who did not exhibit behavioral problems as a child. But, conversely, not all children with behavior problems will carry these into adulthood. Nonetheless, the need for early intervention is critical to prevent progressive decline in behavior.

Like many behavioral problems, disruptive behavior disorders span a continuum ranging from a normal developmental variation, to a problem, to a disorder. These disorders include aggression, Oppositional Defiant Disorder (ODD), Conduct Disorder (CD), antisocial behavior, and delinquency. A high percentage of children show some indicators of externalizing behavioral problems, but the degree of severity causes them to be considered subthreshold or subclinical.

AGGRESSION

Aggression is defined as acts that inflict bodily or mental harm on others. It is the most stable of all early detectable personality characteristics. Normal behavior can include aggression in young children, and ages 2–4 years are peak times for the incidence of aggression. As a result, high false positive rates in diagnosis may occur at younger ages. Typical preschoolers disobey 25%–50% of their parents' commands, and approximately 25% of toddlers are felt to be aggressive. Aggressive behavior can be socially accepted. This is most evident in sports where aggression and violence can take the form of "trash talk" or a "killer instinct". Aggression, at the extreme, can also be antisocial. While almost all aggressive children are oppositional, only some oppositional children are physically aggressive.

VIOLENCE

Violence is aggressive behavior that causes serious harm, while *delinquency* is a legal term used in children arrested for antisocial behavior. It is also used as a clinical descriptive label for these behaviors. *Personality traits* are enduring patterns of behavior that do not reach the threshold for personality disorder.

OPPOSITIONAL DEFIANT DISORDER (ODD)/ CONDUCT DISORDER (CD)

At the extreme of the externalizing continuum are Oppositional Defiant Disorders (ODDs) and Conduct Disorders (CDs) (American Psychiatric Association, 1994). ODD occurs in 2%–16% of the population before the age of 8 years, with modal prevalence rates being 6%–8%. This disorder is characterized by stubbornness, resistance, verbal aggression, disobedience, and a generally difficult temperament. The symptoms are less severe than those found in CD. ODD is also more common in families with a parent who has a mood disorder, attention deficit hyperactivity disorder, antisocial personality disorder, or substance abuse. Symptoms include the following (Diagnostic and Statistical Manual of Mental Disorders-IV; American Psychiatric Association, 1994):

A pattern of negativistic, hostile, defiant behavior lasting at least 6 months and in which four or more of the following are present. The child often:

- Loses his or her temper
- Argues with adults
- Actively defies/refuses to comply with adults' requests/rules
- Deliberately annoys people
- Blames others for his/her mistakes/misbehavior
- Is touchy or easily annoyed by others

- Is angry and resentful
- Is spiteful or vindictive

The behavior occurs more frequently than is typical for the child's age and developmental level, and the impairment is clinically significant. Some researchers argue for a reduction in the number of criteria (i.e., <4) so as to better capture children who need intervention (probably reflecting a position that is a few notches down on the continuum). On a more positive note, ODDs appear to be more amenable to intervention than are CDs.

In contrast, CDs are more serious and more persistent. The estimated prevalence rate is 6%–16% in males and 2%–9% in females younger than 18 years of age. This disorder can occur as early as 5–6 years of age, but the usual onset is late childhood/early adolescence. The onset is earlier in males with a concomitant diagnosis of ADHD (usually before age 12). It is estimated that more than 80% of children with a new diagnosis of CD had a previous diagnosis of oppositional defiant disorder.

DSM-IV criteria (American Psychiatric Association, 1994) define CD as a repetitive and consistent pattern of behavior in which the basic rights of others or major age-appropriate societal norms/rules are violated. Three or more of the following criteria (individual items within the four groups listed below) must be met in the last 12 months, with one or more occurring in the past 6 months:

- *Aggression to people/animals:* (bullies, threatens, intimidates others; initiates physical fights; has used a weapon; physically cruel to people; physically cruel to animals; has stolen while confronting the victim; forced someone into sexual activity)
- *Destruction of property (vandalism):* (deliberately engaged in firesetting; deliberately destroyed others' property)
- *Deceitfulness or theft:* (broken into house, building, car; lies to obtain goods, favors, or avoid obligations; stolen items without confronting victim)
- *Serious violations of rules (status offenses):* (stays out all night [before 13 years of age]; has run away from home overnight more than 2 times; often truant from school [before 13 years]).

CD can be mild, moderate or severe. There is a childhood onset type (10 years or younger) or an adolescent onset type (11 years or older). Again, there has to be clinically significant impairment. There typically is more aggression in children who meet the diagnostic criteria at earlier ages. It is thought that children with CD who are impulsive/hostile/ affective are different from those who are controlled/instrumental/ predatory; children with the former constellation are more emotional and often have ADHD, while behaviors arising from the latter behavioral type are more premeditated and typically occur without remorse.

Relationship between Oppositional-Defiant and Conduct Disorders

The literature supports a distinction between ODD and CD, although ODD is a risk factor for conduct disorder. The presence of ADHD plus an oppositional defiant disorder increases the likelihood of later CD. Interestingly, with respect to *comorbidity* (presence of more than one disorder), 21%–35% of children with ODD *do not have* a comorbid disorder, while 30%–45% of those with CD *do not have* another concomitant diagnosis. Therefore, with respect to ODD, a child has a higher probability of having an additional, "comorbid" disorder, than having ODD in isolation.

A difficult or oppositional temperament, lack of behavioral inhibition, and callousness (lack of sympathy for others, selfishness, diminished guilt) are risk factors that increase the probability of ODD or CD. Family risk factors include low socioeconomic status, poor maternal psychiatric adjustment, criminality in family members, marital discord, divorce, lack of parental involvement/supervision, and harsh or inconsistent punishment. Gender differences in DBD do not emerge until age 6 years or later, with males having higher rates subsequently. In general, the male/female ratio of ODD is fairly equal, while aggression is found more in males. The relationship among ODD, CD, ADHD, and later antisocial personality disorder (which cannot be diagnosed before age 18) is indicated below (see Loeber & Stouthamer-Loeber, 1998).

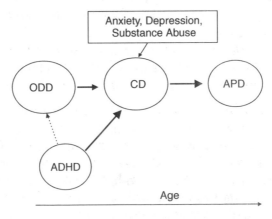

Developmental Sequence

DEVELOPMENTAL SUBTYPES OF AGGRESSION

There are two developmental subtypes of aggression/violent behavior (Moffitt, 1993; Moffitt et al., 1996; Patterson & Yoerger, 1997).

Life-Course Persistent/Early Starters

The *Life Course Persistent/Early Starters* typically demonstrate problem behaviors beginning in the 4–8 year age range. While these children comprise 5%–8% of the population, they account for 50% of later, adolescent crimes. Onset is early, and the younger the age, the greater the severity. These children frequently have so-called neuropsychological vulnerabilities (ADHD, executive dysfunction, communication disorders, slow at learning), and often have parents who, because of their own issues, display disrupted parenting. There is an evocative child-parent interaction, in which aversive child behavior evokes a distinctive parental response, and this occurs in a circular manner. It is estimated that 50% of children who demonstrate these problems before age 11 continue past age 20; the more severe, the greater the likelihood of persistence.

Adolescent-Limited/Late Onset

The second subtype is the *Adolescent Limited/Late Onset Type* (Moffitt, 1993; Moffitt et al., 1996; Patterson & Yoerger, 1997). It is postulated that there is a discrepancy between biologic and social age or a gap between biological maturity and social maturity in these older children/adolescents. Essentially, the adolescent is physiologically advanced but socially restricted. As a result, these individuals engage in "social mimicry" where they learn from the aforementioned life-course persistent models. The life-course persistent adolescents are idolized because they typically have more possessions, are sexually experienced, free from families of origin, often have fathered children, and have their own attorney, social worker, or probation officer. The disruptive behavior in those who demonstrate the later, adolescent limited externalizing disorders, does not occur across situations (only when it is profitable) and the peak age of occurrence is approximately 17 years of age. These adolescents are not as alienated from their families and typically desist in this behavior by young adulthood.

Hence the developmental course of disruptive behavior disorders is multiply-determined and best considered transactional. This conceptualization is demonstrated below. Basically, there are child components (upper two left and center boxes), environmental risks (bottom left circle), parenting issues (bottom right oval), and child behaviors (upper right box) that contribute to the emergence, severity, and persistence of DBDs. All components must be considered by the practitioner.

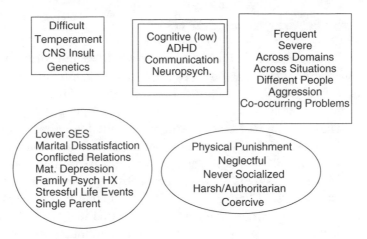

Risks for Disruptive Disorders (Transactional)

PROTECTIVE FACTORS

Conversely, there are protective factors that tend to lower the probability of disruptive behavior disorders, or the persistence of these disorders. These factors include: (1) family support (immediate and extended members), (2) schools that promote active involvement of family and focus on positive school adjustment, achievement and prosocial behavior, (3) positive community socialization (tutoring, mentoring, modeling), and (4) mastery of coping competence (affective, social, and achievement). With respect to treatment, there are several basic tenets: (1) intervention must be early, (2) key family and social risk as well as protective factors must be targeted, (3) coping competence must be promoted, (4) academic success must be fostered, and (5) early on, the focus should be on promoting optimal parenting styles and parent-child interactions, particularly in the 4–8 year age range. It has been reported that if parents are instructed about these practices, 30%–40% will continue. Improved social skills in children are associated with decreased aggression.

ASSESSMENT FRAMEWORK

If the practitioner is presented with the task of assessing a child with externalizing problems, the following framework is recommended (see Frick & O'Brien, 1995):

I. Classification	ODD/CD/normal developmental variation
	Socialized/under-socialized behavior
	Aggressive/non-aggressive
	Early onset/late onset
	Instrumental/reactive
II. Comorbidities	ADHD
	Anxiety/depression
	Learning disabilities/cognitive limitations
	Communication disorders
	Neuropsychological issues (executive dysfunction; poor social awareness)
III. Correlates	Family functioning
	Social ecology
	Peer relations

Consideration of the child's emotional reactivity, response to discipline, degree of aggressiveness, and behavioral impulsivity is necessary. The Child Behavior Checklist (CBCL; Achenbach, 1991), Personality Inventory for Children-2 (PIC-2, Lachar & Gruber, 2001), Behavior Assessment System for Children (BASC; Reynolds & Kamphaus, 1992) or the Eyeberg Child Behavior Inventory (ECBI; Eyberg,1999) are useful instruments. The Children's Aggression Scale-P (CAS-P; Halperin et al., 2002) provides questions that are highly informative and can be incorporated into the clinical interview. Items contained in this instrument specifically target the frequency, severity, and location (within/outside home environment) of true aggression.

SUMMARY

In summary, disruptive, externalizing disorders represent the extreme of the problem behavior continuum. They also demonstrate the complexity in the relationships among child, environmental, and interactive factors that influence the development of problem behaviors. How these variables interrelate will determine the severity of the problem, and this matrix helps to explain individual differences. These behaviors have a major, negative impact on the child's self-concept, interpersonal relations, and the eventual developmental paths that the child follows.

The following chapters of this text will address how the practitioner and parents may intervene to prevent the emergence of these more serious behaviors.

Chapter 5

Theories and Practice

Appreciation of the major conceptual frameworks of developmental theory is important both in terms of defining a behavioral problem and providing models for intervention (Simeonsson & Rosenthal, 1999). The best overall approach that is used to treat behavioral problems must be pragmatic and eclectic, but it should contain strong behavioral underpinnings. That said, it is valuable for the practitioner to be aware of the major premises of the most prominent developmental models. Because in-depth discussion of these developmental theories is beyond the scope of this book, a brief overview is provided.

MATURATIONAL THEORY

The major premise of this theory (Gesell et al., 1940) is that development reflects a predetermined unfolding of events, and this unfolding is determined by the child's genetic structure and expression. Therefore, behavior is determined and heavily influenced by both neurological and physical maturation. While one's genetic endowment and its resultant influence on physical and neurological development unequivocally influences behavior, this theoretic approach neglects to acknowledge the powerful effects of environmental, social, and cognitive (learning) processes.

PSYCHODYNAMIC MODEL

This model, originated by Freud, and refined by Klein (1958) and Anna Freud (1963), is often considered *psychoanalytic* or *psychosexual*. The system is biologically-based and the principal tenet is that development is affected by a continuous drive to gratify basic needs that arise from infancy through adolescence. As a result, this approach is designed to explain personality and behavior. Early experiences that are either too stressful or overly enjoyable are thought to influence later behaviors in an unacknowledged (unconscious) manner. The interaction between the child and parent(s) is a crucial factor and will influence the development of the child's personality and his ability to adjust and adapt to different situations.

There is a series of psychosexual stages that the child progresses through: oral [birth to 18 months], anal [18 months to 3 years], phallic [3–6 years], latency [6–11 years], and genital [adolescence–adulthood]. This progression, with development of the id, ego, and superego, determines one's personality and emotional development. Major developmental acquisitions of each stage, respectively, include: oral pleasure, control of bodily functions, sex-role identification, repression of sexuality, and renewed heterosexual interest.

Problems are thought to arise from the failure to gratify needs appropriately, resulting in persistence of these behaviors in later ages (*fixation*) or a tendency to return to earlier stages of development when stressed (*regression*). This model is useful because of its emphasis on the mother-child interaction, and the tripartite conceptualization of the personality: *id* (storehouse for instinctual energy, driven by the "pleasure principle"), *ego* (rational, reality-oriented component of the personality, based on the "reality principle"), and *superego* (moral/ethical part of the personality). Concomitant defense mechanisms also are useful in conceptualizing problem behavior. Self-concept results from the resolution of conflicts between the child's inner needs and social demands. The defense mechanisms of *denial* (not acknowledging or being aware of a stressful situation when one exists) and *projection* (unknowingly attributing one's feelings and motivations to another) are particularly prevalent in childhood.

It stands to reason that early experiences influence adult behaviors and motivations to a significant degree, and these early experiences would have a major impact on subsequent parenting behaviors as well. Moreover, the various permutations of the child's needs, parent-child interaction, and the balance between needs and external demands help to explain the uniqueness of individuals. Interpersonal experiences with an affective load are central to personality development and the development of the capacity to develop and maintain subsequent emotional relationships. This truly underscores the vital role the family has on healthy emotional development.

PSYCHOSOCIAL MODEL

This theoretic orientation expands the psychoanalytic approach to include environmental/psychosocial influences on the healthy development of the personality (ego). More specifically, Erikson (1963) places much emphasis on early development, particularly the period of infancy (and the mother-child interaction), as well as societal influences. Each of eight stages of ego development (five are applicable from infancy through adolescence) is characterized by a psychosocial crisis or so-called nuclear conflict in which the child essentially must balance opposing forces such as: (1) *trust versus mistrust*, (2) *autonomy versus shame and doubt*, (3) *initiative versus guilt*, (4) *industry versus inferiority*, (5) *identity versus identity diffusion* and so on. Resolution of the crises reflects meeting the needs of the ego in the context of socialization. In sequence from infancy through adolescence, the stages involve: (a) receipt of social support, (b) independence, (c) self-care, (d) social skills, and (e) definition of self. By resolving each of the nuclear conflicts, the child has to develop in sequence: trust and a sense of dependability regarding the external world; self-control without a loss of self-esteem; ambition, independence and self-confidence; satisfaction emanating from achievement, recognition, and success; and a feeling of comfort with one's sense of self. Failure to resolve a conflict at earlier ages will destabilize the hierarchical developmental progression; however, this is a lifespan model, and as such the possibility of change at later ages is acknowledged. For example, although in the Trust versus Mistrust stage the experiences of the first year of life will strongly influence the child's attitude about dependability regarding the outside world, "disruption" can be repaired over time by other, more positive aspects of the social environment. The model is clinically useful in that it considers the child's developmental stage and its related issues (e.g., need for nurturance, independence, challenge, sense of self), and how the environment responds to these issues (e.g., provision of nurturance, restrictiveness, encouragement, conformity) in the evolution of emotional/social-interactive development. The radius of environmental/ social influences expands sequentially from maternal figure → paternal figure → family → neighborhood and schools → peer groups.

COGNITIVE MODEL

Piaget's theory was discussed briefly in Chapter 3 (Piaget & Inhelder, 1969). The basic premise is that the child is intrinsically motivated to make sense out of the environment and in so doing, actively experiences and interacts with the environment. Emerging physical and mental capacities are used to actively engage the environment. The child's understanding of the environment and cognitive development are directly related to how he or she *experiences* the environment. Assimilation and accommodation enable adaptation, and the child proceeds through a series of stages in which the rate varies, but the sequence is invariant (sensorimotor period {birth to 2 years}; preoperational period {2–7 years}; concrete operations {7–11 years}; and formal operations {11–15 years}). Major developmental acquisitions in the sensorimotor period include development of object permanence, sense of causality, appreciation of spatial relationships, and use of instruments. In the preoperational period, (in addition to the cognitive characteristics mentioned previously such as egocentricity, animism, etc.), early reasoning emerges. By the concrete operational stage, "conservation" (ability to have cognitive representations essentially override perceptions—that is, reasoning supercedes appearances), and deductive reasoning occur. By the stage of formal operations, there is development of abstract ideas and concepts, inductive reasoning, the ability to generate multiple hypotheses as to what caused a given situation, and to the capacity to connect future consequences to a current behavior (thereby allowing the child to give informed consent, versus assent).

An imbalance (disequilibrium) between assimilation and accommodation provides the basis for maladaption; assimilation is considered *organizational* (incorporating the environment into existing cognitive structures), while accommodation reflects *coping* (adjusting cognitive structures to the environment). Both work in unison to enable the child to make sense of the world. Perhaps the most extreme example of excessive emphasis on assimilation is autistic-like thought, exemplified by impairments in the so-called "theory of mind" (appreciation of the mental states/processes of others). Play is considered to be pure assimilation, while imitation is pure accommodation. The ability to accommodate is critical for information acquisition. Maturation and experience influence cognitive development, and the child's manner of thinking will influence how she might experience the world, and how her behaviors will influence those around her. Perhaps the most important message from the cognitive developmental theories is that we must realize that children think in a manner that is qualitatively different from adults. Many cognitive characteristics (discussed in Chapter 3) produce behaviors that might otherwise seem unusual, unless the parent understands the underlying explanations for such behavior.

Moral Development

Related to this is Kohlberg's (1964) theory of moral development in which moral reasoning proceeds through three levels, each containing two stages. Early on, rules are obeyed to get rewards and avoid punishment;

hence consequences of actions are important. Driving forces are external to the self versus internalized (preconventional morality). Subsequently, children obey rules and social norms in order to win others' approval. Praise and avoidance of blame are now important. Actions are evaluated by the person's intent, not necessarily the outcome. Prior to approximately 10 to 11 years of age, there exists moral absolutism in which fixed rules are adhered to in a rigid fashion, as long as they are imposed by a legitimate authority. With increasing age and cognitive development, the child develops a more relative understanding of right and wrong, and the capacity for more abstract thought.

BEHAVIORAL MODEL

This theoretic approach addresses overt behavior and not psychological or developmental underpinnings per se. Stated differently, functional aspects of behavior are prime foci, with little attention being paid to developmental issues (Kazdin, 1975; Skinner, 1953). Emphasis is on observable phenomena or behavior, not motives. It is assumed that the child's past reinforcement history has contributed to current behaviors; these behaviors, however, are not necessarily considered symptomatic of underlying conflicts or developmental transitions.

This orientation differs from the medical model mindset. In the medical model, an internal, underlying condition such as a bacterial infection will produce the symptoms of vomiting or fever. The remedy would be to treat the cause of the problem (bacterial infection) and not just the symptoms. However, under the strict behavioral model, if a child is excessively aggressive, the practitioner will focus on treating the aggressive behavior itself, and not be concerned with the underlying cause or reasons that influenced the behavior. Moreover, it is assumed that once behavior is changed, cognitive and affective alterations will follow.

The child's behavior is broken down into simple elements that can be related to specific stimuli or contingencies. Intervention is directed to current, versus past, conditions. Behavior is learned by imitation, observation, or associations, and it is rewarded or reinforced in some manner. This learning can become more complex by the evolution of forward or backward chains of association, thereby sometimes making it difficult to identify the initial antecedents and consequences of the behavior. There are three types of learning that are involved in the behavioral approach: (1) *Classical conditioning*, (2) *Operant conditioning*, and (3) *Social learning/modeling*. Each will be discussed below.

Classical Conditioning

This type of learning is also called *respondent conditioning, stimulus-stimulus learning* or *Pavlovian conditioning*. The first premise is that certain stimuli cause particular responses without any prior learning. For example, onions cause tearing, or an unexpected, loud noise will produce a startle. In this "automatic" association, the stimulus (onion, loud noise) is called the *unconditioned stimulus* (UCS) and the response (tearing, startle) is the *unconditioned response* (UCR). In classical conditioning, the second necessary component is that a previously neutral stimulus (one that would not initially elicit an "automatic" response) is temporally paired with the UCS (stimulus that normally would elicit the response). After such pairing (usually several times) the previously neutral stimulus (*conditioned stimulus*; CS) will elicit the same response that the UCS had done previously (the response to the conditioned stimulus is now called the *conditioned response*—CR).

Examples of Classical Conditioning

This paradigm is sometimes called Pavlovian conditioning because it was first reported by Ivan Pavlov in his work with dogs. Briefly, in Pavlov's work, presentation of meat powder (UCS) produced salivation (UCR). In a serendipitous temporal pairing, a factory bell (CS) rang immediately prior to presentation of the meat powder, and after several pairings, presentation of the bell then produced salivation (CR) in the absence of meat powder. This is shown graphically below.

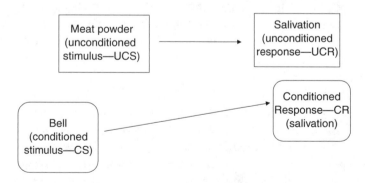

Example of Classical Conditioning

Another example involves the case of a 4-year-old child who sneaks out of the house and suddenly sees a *squirrel* in a tree that he finds cute and interesting (CS; conditioned stimulus). Just as the child approaches the squirrel, a nearby garbage truck has a major *backfire* (UCS; unconditioned stimulus) causing a fearful *startle reaction* in the child (UCR; unconditioned response), who then runs back into the house, screaming. The next time the child goes out of the house with his mother, he again sees a squirrel (CS; conditioned stimulus), and becomes fearful, screaming and struggling to go back into the house (CR; conditioned response). Via chaining, or second-order conditioning, the child subsequently cries when he approaches the front door before leaving the house. It becomes obvious how the emergence of this fear response could be totally perplexing to the child's parents, especially if they were unaware of the initial incident. Similarly, if a child consumed a novel food, or even a favorite dessert, but then became sick and vomited, it is highly probable that the child would avoid this food on subsequent occasions (the associative chain being food → vomiting → malaise).

A familiar, seminal example of classical conditioning in children is found in the case of Little Albert (Watson & Rayner, 1920). Watson was interested in fear responses of children and investigated this in an infant who came from a local orphanage. Initially, Albert was not fearful of furry things such as cotton, a rabbit, a white rat (ubiquitous in psychology), or a dog. However, the youngster was readily frightened by loud noises (produced by hitting a suspended metal bar with a hammer behind Albert's head). The respondent conditioning procedure then consisted of showing Albert the white rat (CS), immediately followed by striking the bar and making a loud noise (UCS) which produced crying (UCR). After several such pairings, presentation of the rat alone (a previously "neutral" stimulus) produced fear and crying (CR). This behavior generalized to a multitude of furry objects, including Santa's white beard.

Counter-Conditioning

Classically conditioned fears can also be reversed or "counter conditioned" using similar techniques. This was demonstrated in the famous case of Peter, who had a phobia of rabbits (Jones, 1924). While it is not clear how this fear developed, in counter-conditioning the rabbit was associated with ice cream and peer modeling, so that the aversion to the rabbit gradually dissipated. This was an "in vivo" approach. This type of procedure is very similar to systematic desensitization (Wolpe, 1958) in which anxiety that is associated with a feared object, person, place or activity is replaced with incompatible relaxation (which is incompatible with tenseness that arises from anxiety). The child is taught to relax various muscle groups, and once relaxed, he mentally visualizes scenes that come closer and closer to the feared object or situation. The mental scenes are extracted from a pre-determined fear or anxiety hierarchy. The goal is to associate the feared object or situation with relaxation, thereby short-circuiting the object-anxiety connection.

Enuresis

The popular alarm method of dealing with enuresis is another example of classical conditioning. This was originally deemed the bell-and-pad method of the 1950's, where the first drops of urine completed a circuit on a metal grid imbedded in a pad underneath the child. This then caused an alarm to ring. Contemporary alarms are much more sophisticated and range from simple inserts that are placed in the child's underwear to watch devices, or radio transmitters. The schematic for this paradigm is found below.

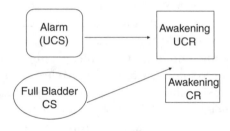

Enuresis Alarm

Basically, the alarm (UCS) routinely produces awakening (UCR). A full bladder (CS) is then associated temporally with the onset of the alarm (due to the release of the initial drops of urine). The full bladder, and its associated pressure, is considered a neutral stimulus, because it is not causing awakening on its own. However, with several pairings of the full bladder with the alarm, the full bladder by itself will cause the child to awaken (CR). Having the child urinate after awakening, and providing some reward the next morning are two additional components of this successful treatment program.

In actuality, many feared mental images or even words are classically conditioned to emotions. For example, when working with a family whose 8-year-old child has pseudoseizures, the problem should be reframed, with the word, "seizure" being termed "the problem" so as to bypass associations with the affect-laden word (seizure) that emerge when the word is mentioned. Similarly, words such as "spider," "monster," or "snake" have affective ties, these typically due to previous conditioning.

In summary, classical or respondent conditioning plays a major part in the development of fears, phobias, school refusal, post-traumatic stress disorders, food aversions, and selective mutism. Similarly, treatment of these conditions involves counter-conditioning of the original temporal associations and anxiety. Real-life "paradigms" are not necessarily pure classical conditioning, because they often include modeling and/or elements of operant conditioning. Classical conditioning also can explain why children are frightened to come to the physician's office, or their fear of white coats; these previously neutral stimuli have become associated with shots, physical examinations or some other stressful procedure, and now are conditioned stimuli in and of themselves.

Operant Conditioning

Operant conditioning is often called *instrumental conditioning*, or *stimulus-response learning*. Corresponding to Pavlov's status in classical conditioning, B.F. Skinner (1953) is considered the original proponent of this approach. The term, operant conditioning, is derived from the fact that the behaviors are considered operants because they *operate* on the environment by causing environmental consequences. The paradigm is best conceptualized as stimulus → response → reinforcement. Antecedent stimuli influence operant behavior by providing a context conducive to its occurrence or its inhibition. Reduced to essential basics, a behavior is analyzed and modified by identifying and manipulating its *antecedents* and *consequences*.

Operant Behavioral Problems

It is safe to say that the majority of behavior problems found in pediatric settings are operant in nature (Hirsch & Russo, 1983). These problems tend to fall into three categories: (a) *behavioral deficiencies* (not doing chores, not doing homework, not staying in the yard, not defecating on the toilet), (b) *behavioral excesses* (tantrums, aggression, disregard of authority), or (c) *behavioral inappropriateness* (breaking objects, urinating on the floor, making frequent, inappropriate statements) (Hirsch & Russo, 1983). This distinction is helpful because some intervention procedures tend to increase the frequency of a desired behavior pattern or the development of a new behavior; other interventions help to decrease the frequency of the behavior or change the time or place of occurrence of the behavior. Procedures that increase or decrease the frequency of behavior tend to focus on consequences that follow the behavior, while procedures that change the time or place of occurrence of a behavior focus on antecedent stimuli that control the behavior. Timing, intensity, and consistency are critical factors in both the development and management of behavioral problems.

Methods of Altering Behaviors

There are four major ways of altering behavior: *positive reinforcement, negative reinforcement, punishment*, and *extinction*. Each will be discussed below. Thorndike's "law of effect" basically holds that behaviors that are followed by positive consequences will have a greater likelihood of reoccurring in the future. Conversely, those behaviors that are not followed by positive consequences will have a decreased likelihood of occurring once again. Hence, what follows the behavior is important. Similarly, the "Premack principle" states that those behaviors which have a low probability of occurrence can be increased by having them be the prerequisite for performance of a higher probability behavior (e.g., eat your carrots and then you can have dessert). Treatment of behavioral problems sometimes falls under the title of *applied behavior analysis*.

Positive Reinforcement.   Positive reinforcement is the process in which there is an increase in the frequency of a specific behavior when it is followed by a favorable or desirable event (Martin & Pear, 1996). If the child, in a given situation, displays a behavior and this behavior is followed immediately by a positive consequence, the same behavior is more likely to be displayed again in the future under similar circumstances. Desirable consequences are referred to as *positive reinforcers* and these can be: (a) edible (candy, gum, ice cream, soda), (b) tangible or manipulative (toy, collectible, computer game), (c) an activity (go to the zoo, playing games, staying up later), or (d) social (praise, hugging). A positive reinforcer is technically different than a reward although they tend to sometimes be used interchangeably. Rewards are things given or received for an achievement of some type; a positive reinforcer is defined by its effect on a behavior, namely, it increases the behavior.

The effectiveness of a positive reinforcer is influenced by whether it is given to the child on a *contingent* basis, namely it is provided only when the child demonstrates a specific, targeted behavior (not inconsistently delivered, and the defined behavior cannot be ambiguous) (Parrish, 1997). For example, if a child is taken on a trip to the local ice cream store because he is "good," even though he might not have been, or the meaning of "good" is not specifically defined, then the effectiveness of the positive reinforcer is attenuated. The child would be less likely to appreciate the fact or make the connection that displaying prosocial behavior leads to a positive consequence. This is true because he is reinforced even if this behavior is not displayed, or the requirements for such behavior are not specified.

Schedules of Reinforcement. The *immediacy* of the positive reinforcement is critical; more immediate reinforcement is more effective in changing behavior than is delayed reinforcement. This is especially the case in younger children who do not possess the cognitive capabilities to maintain the association among a behavior and a reinforcement for a long period of time. Perhaps most critical is the *schedule of reinforcement*. Positive reinforcement can be provided after a certain number of responses have occurred (*ratio schedule*) or after passage of a certain amount of time relative to the child's performance (*interval schedule*). These schedules can be fixed or variable. *Fixed schedules* occur after a specific number of responses are produced by the child, or after a consistent amount of time has lapsed (with the next response being reinforced). In real-life situations where problems develop, *variable schedules* are typical, particularly the variable ratio schedule. A child may receive a positive reinforcement on one occasion after asking her mother for candy once, while on other occasions it might be as much as ten times before the candy is forthcoming. The point is that the child does not know which time the behavior will be followed by a positive reinforcement and hence will keep trying, anticipating that the next response will be reinforced. This type of parental behavior is often termed *inconsistency*, and it makes the child's behavior problems very resistant to intervention. In fact, variable ratio reinforcement is the basic principle involved in slot machines or lotteries.

A variable interval situation might have the problem behaviors occur over an extended amount of time, with the parent finally offering a concession to the next response that the child emits. Positive reinforcement dispensed on a variable ratio schedule could explain why a child keeps coming up with excuses so he can stay up later at bedtime (staying up being the positive reinforcement), or a child in a supermarket who keeps wheedling his mother to purchase a small toy and is subsequently given the toy to "shut him up." Continuous reinforcement (essentially a fixed ratio schedule) occurs when the child is reinforced each and every time a behavior is displayed. This approach is often used in the beginning of a positive reinforcement schedule to increase the likelihood of a desired response, and can subsequently be reduced in a gradual manner.

Unfortunately, sometimes reprimands, holding a child tightly on one's lap to keep her in time out, or yelling at a child constantly can be positive reinforcers, particularly if the child is seeking attention (whether it be positive or negative). One must remember that parental attention is an extremely potent reinforcer (in fact, referring back to classical conditioning, maternal attention is sometimes considered an unconditioned stimulus). Reprimands are highly reinforcing to a child who does not otherwise receive attention. "Giving in" to behaviors such as whining, pouting, or crying are examples of positive reinforcement unintentionally increasing less desirable behavior.

The *uniqueness* of the reinforcement is critical, and often the most effective reinforcement could be directly related to the issue at hand. More specifically, if a child is desirous of the mother's attention because of the birth of a new sibling, and engages in problem behaviors as a means of getting the mother's attention, then maternal attention can be used as a positive reinforcer for more appropriate behavior. Similarly, *satiation* and *deprivation* play a role. If the child has 20 videogames and the reinforcement for appropriate behavior is yet another, similar game, then the efficacy is reduced. However, if the child has not played games for quite some time (but is highly eager to do so) or has only one or two games, and now is able to earn a new game, this reinforcement is much more effective. This scenario often occurs in the use of monetary reinforcers. The impact of accumulating money is vitiated by the fact that parents give the child spending money for activities such as going to the movies, regardless of the behavioral program that is put in place. Hence there is less of a need for the earned monetary reward. Novel reinforcers are typically more effective when they are first introduced.

Positive reinforcers can be *primary* (food, hugs, something tangible that the child wants) or *secondary* (stickers, tokens, coupons, checks). A key issue is the fact that secondary reinforcers need to be tied into something primary, otherwise they will rapidly become ineffective. At its extreme, the use of "untied" secondary reinforcers is analogous to an adult being given Monopoly money for a job well done. This is seen in real-life situations in which a child is repeatedly given stickers on a calendar for good behavior but the stickers are not tied into (or redeemed for) some other type of tangible reinforcement. Instead, a ratio schedule (e.g., three stickers equals a trip to a fast food restaurant) would be much more productive in terms of changing behaviors. Tokens, grades, happy faces from the teacher, and so on are additional secondary reinforcers that are used frequently.

Negative Reinforcement.   Negative reinforcement refers to facilitating an increase in the frequency of a response by removing an unpleasant or aversive stimulus, immediately after the response is performed. When removed, the behavior that preceded the negative reinforcer tends to *increase* in frequency. Basically, the child works to have the negative reinforcer taken away. Negative reinforcement is frequently misconstrued as being a punishment, which it is not. The key difference is that removal of negative reinforcement *increases* the behavior that it follows; presentation of punishment *decreases* the behavior that precedes it. Negative reinforcement occurs frequently in day-to-day routines. For example, a child will eventually wear a coat on a cold day to avoid the aversive state of being cold. A person buckles a seatbelt to have to buzzer turn off, while a student in class will pay attention so that the teacher will stop reminding her to do so in front of the entire class. Cold, the irritating buzzer noise, and the teacher's reminders are negative reinforcers.

Positive and Negative Reinforcement in Combination. A combination of positive and negative reinforcement often occurs in problematic parent-child interactions (Parrish, 1999; Hirsch & Russo, 1983). For example, if the child wanted to watch a video, but the parents were viewing the evening news on the television, the child may cry, whine, or complain loudly. This behavior would persist for some time, and the parents then might finally give in and allow the child to put the video on. In this type of interaction, the parent's behavior is *negatively reinforced*, because it appeases the child and causes him to stop the negative, annoying behavior. Conversely, the child's behavior, because it leads to a desired outcome, is *positively reinforced*.

Stated differently, the child receives positive reinforcement for whining and crying, while the termination of this aversive behavior is a negative reinforcement for the parents. Had the child's behavior led to a time-out instead, this would have then been a punishment. Negative reinforcement occurs in the aforementioned "coercive" parent-child interactions, when a child's misbehavior is followed by yelling, screaming, or verbal threats from the parents. In order to avoid the aversive parental behaviors, the child's behaviors become more compliant (and hence lead to the cessation of the negative reinforcer).

As a result, negative reinforcement typically leads to *escape* or *avoidance behavior*. Avoidance behavior prevents the onset of a negative reinforcement by the child making a response; escape behavior occurs when a negative reinforcement is turned off or terminated by performance of an action. In an example of an avoidance situation, a child may fear going to the playground at recess, because other children make fun of him and sometimes are verbally aggressive. Rather than go out at recess (preferring to stay alone in the classroom), the child may not complete his work in the classroom and therefore have to remain inside at recess to complete it. The negative reinforcer here is peer ridicule/aggression, and the behavior that prevents its occurrence is not completing classwork (thereby causing the child to remain inside and avoid the playground). Had the child been sent to the playground and then complained of a headache in order to go back into the school building, this would be an escape situation (the unpleasant stimulus, peer ridicule/aggression, is experienced but then terminated by leaving the playground). Interestingly, avoidance behavior is more durable or long-lasting than escape behavior, as the child will work very hard to not experience the negative reinforcer in any manner. Moreover, the anticipation and fear of the negative rein-forcer are in some cases worse than actually experiencing it.

Punishment.   Punishment occurs when an unpleasant consequence follows a behavior, or a positive reinforcer is withdrawn contingent on the performance of a behavior (Martin & Pear, 1996). The end result is a decrease in the probability of that behavior occurring again in the future. Hence there are two components to punishment: (1) a behavior is imme-diately followed by an undesirable consequence, and (2) the child is less likely to engage in the behavior again in similar situations (i.e., the frequency of the behavior is decreased). The undesirable consequence of the behavior is called a *punisher*.

Punishment is not necessarily mean, painful, or hurtful, but, unfortu-nately it can be so at times, if it is misapplied. As such, punishment is controversial, and in practice, the term, "consequences," is better applied. As mentioned previously, punishment teaches a child what *not* to do, but does not necessarily incorporate the other aspect of the overall approach of discipline, namely, also teaching a child what *to* do. In general, parents and professionals prefer to use positive reinforcement strategies first. Even if punishment is then employed, continuation of positive reinforce-ment to foster a more desirable, competing response is also necessary, so as to enhance learning of more appropriate behaviors. Unfortunately, some caretakers immediately resort to punishment tactics as a means of control-ling behavior, without giving much thought to positive reinforcement (which is sometimes considered to be "bribery"). These same households also often employ corporal punishment as the primary punisher.

Corporal Punishment.   Corporal punishment involves spanking, hitting, or other physical means to cause the child to stop a behavior. It is highly controversial, and is driven by cultural norms, parent charac-teristics and beliefs, child characteristics, and contextual effects such as momentary outbursts of anger (e.g., Strauss, 1994). It is estimated that 90% of parents spank 3-year-olds; 60% of 10- to 12-year-olds are struck. Parents who believe that this type of punishment is acceptable typically believe in strict discipline, are conservative, over-interpret the seriousness of the transgression (seeing it as being intentional and the child having the ability to control the behavior), and are unable to quickly generate alternative disciplinary responses (Holden, Miller, & Harris, 1999). This type of punishment is generally ineffective for several reasons. First, use of physical force puts the child in danger of injury, and it is difficult to draw a line between a "swat" and a more injurious blow. Moreover, a bruise left on a child mandates reporting. Second, to be effective, physical punishment must be harsh or intense, again raising the possibility of injury. In general, painful punishments have to be increased to maintain effectiveness. Third, there is minimal learning involved, with the behavior simply being suppressed by the child. Fourth, aggression is modeled or imitated by children, and the message implied is that aggression is acceptable. Spanking is also associated with more critical verbalizations which themselves further demean the child. Fifth, parents actually are more inconsistent with respect to corporal punishment, in that they typically might tell a child to stop the problematic behavior several times, becoming increasingly angry in the process. Eventually, after many warnings and intensified anger, the parent loses control, explodes, and physically punishes the child—after the child had essentially gotten away with the misbehavior on at least several occasions in the chain of events. To further decrease the efficacy of the punishment, the parent may subsequently feel guilty about the behavior and then become overly indulgent, thereby, in actuality, reinforcing the problem behavior that initiated the sequence of events in the first place. Sixth, punishment frequently leads to effects that are specific to situations in which the response is punished and to the person who is doing the punishing. As a result, these effects can be very short term and not persistent (leading to so-called "response recovery"). Finally, there simply are better ways of controlling behavior.

Practitioners should be aware that they might encounter resistance to discontinuation of corporal punishment in some parents who have experienced corporal punishment in their own upbringing. The practitioner, in simply stating that physical punishment is not good often is not persuasive and will be summarily discounted unless the claim is supported by other information (e.g., that listed above) and alternative techniques to address the behavior are provided.

Punishment in general, and corporal punishment in particular, can produce emotional sequelae such as crying, fearfulness, anxiety, anger, depression, and aggression. People or situations can be associated with the punishment per se and become a "conditioned punisher" along the lines of conditioning noted previously. Parents who resort to physical punishment often are negatively reinforced for this behavior, as the annoying behavior of the child is suppressed. Hence they are more likely to use it in the future.

Therefore, it is recommended that punishment not be the first line of intervention in dealing with a problem behavior. If it indeed has to be employed, then removal of positive events, and loss of privileges are the most useful consequences. Time out and logical consequences (to be discussed subsequently) are particularly effective techniques.

Differential Reinforcement of Incompatible Behavior (DRI). This technique is used to decrease undesirable behavior by reinforcing a competing behavior that is more desirable. For example, if the problem involves the child picking his fingernails, the child is reinforced for keeping his hands on the desk, thereby preventing the non-desirable behavior from occurring. Similarly, if a youngster sucks her fingers in the classroom, the teacher might set up an agreement that when she sees the child with her hands folded on the desk, she will discretely place a paperclip in a jar. A certain number of paperclips could then be redeemed for a reward.

Extinction. Extinction causes cessation of a response by withholding reinforcement for a response that had previously been reinforced. Basically, the child had displayed a behavior that paid off, but now does not receive this reinforcement. This results in a decreased likelihood that the behavior will occur in similar situations. Extinction is analogous to "ignoring" the behavior, and is one of the most frequent bits of advice given by practitioners to parents. In actuality, it is "planned ignoring" because the caretaker is ignoring the behavior in a predetermined, consistent fashion. This type of intervention is routinely applied when the child nags, whines, cries, has temper tantrums, or displays bedtime refusal.

Extinction is most effective if paired with use of positive reinforcement for a more desirable, competing response, or if followed by a negative consequence. Parents need to be aware that an initial attempt at extinction will often be met by an *increase* in the frequency and intensity of the undesirable behavior. Basically, the child is anticipating that persistence will pay off or lead to the desired reinforcement and he therefore demonstrates a so-called *extinction burst* (meaning that things could get a lot worse before they get better). In actuality, the appearance of an extinction burst paradoxically is an indicator that the intervention is on the right track and is having an impact. This potential increase in problem behavior necessitates implementation of an extinction program on a weekend or at a time when both parents are available (or when a single parent might have some backup or ample time to initiate the program). Consistency is critical, lest the partial reinforcement schedule noted previously come into play. Parents also need to be prepared for the possible re-emergence of the behavior after it has been extinguished, even without any apparent reinforcement. This is called *spontaneous recovery* and the danger is that the behavior might unwittingly be reinforced and hence start the entire cycle once again.

For example, assume a child whines for a treat prior to dinner, and previously she was reinforced 50% of the time because the parent was busy and giving in was easier than listening to the relentless whining. With extinction, the parent first needs to tell the child that she absolutely will not receive a snack prior to dinner and that whining about it will not get her the snack. If the child then continues to do so, reminding her one time is ample (with the addition of telling her that she must leave the room if it continues), and the parent(s) must steadfastly not give in. The child will most likely whine even more initially, in an aforementioned extinction burst. While simply ignoring the behavior would indeed work, the process of engaging in the whining behavior itself might be reinforcing to the child. This is where concomitant use of a consequence or a positive reinforcement is helpful. With the former, the child would be required to also leave the kitchen if she continues to whine; with the latter, the child is told she can definitely have a treat after dinner, if the whining subsides.

Using a metaphor, extinction of a behavior such as a temper tantrum (designed to get attention) would be analogous to having a child on a stage. The curtain rises, but now there is no audience to view the tantrum. However, going through the tantrum on stage might be reinforcing in and of itself. A better technique would be to have the curtain go up without an audience, and as soon as the child begins the tantrum, he is removed from the stage (vis à vis the Gong Show), and immediately placed in a corner for a time out.

In general, a variable ratio schedule is hardest to extinguish. Extinction is most rapid if the behavior was initially established with a continuous reinforcement schedule.

Shaping. Shaping refers to the gradual development of a new behavior, in which positive reinforcement is delivered in response to small improvements in the child's behavior, that get closer and closer to a desired behavior. This is also termed *successive approximations*. This type of behavioral intervention was first described in experimental animal work, in which a rat was placed in a box, and if the animal simply looked at the lever that dispenses food pellets, the experimenter released a pellet. The next step would be to have the animal approach the lever to merit a reinforcement, then approach it more closely, until finally the animal would have to press the lever in order to receive the pellet. This technique often is utilized real-life situations such as with a child who demonstrates selective mutism. The first reinforcement might be delivered contingent upon the child looking at the therapist. The next step would be to reward the child for nodding or shaking her head in response to questions poised by the therapist. Reinforcement would subsequently be contingent upon the child making some sound in conjunction with the gesture, next an actual word, and then a string of words. This procedure can also be used to address feeding disorders, toileting problems, or the child sleeping in the parents' bed.

Less desirable behaviors can also evolve by means of shaping. For example, a child may first come into the parents' bed in response to a storm. The next time the child wakes up during the night, he may simply wander into the bed, unbeknownst to the sleeping parents. Eventually, this could evolve into the child insisting that he go to sleep in the parents' bed at the beginning of the bedtime ritual. In this, as well as other similar situations, the onset of the problem is insidious and often it is not identified as a problem until the behavior has become extreme.

Fading.   Fading occurs when the positive reinforcer is withdrawn slowly, while the desired, newly learned behavior continues. Essentially, in day-to-day application, the positive reinforcement becomes less frequent. For example, assume the child is allowed to obtain a grab-bag every time a star is received for sitting on the toilet. Once the behavior is regularly displayed, access to the grab-bag may necessitate receipt of two stars, then three stars, and so on. Fading often occurs "naturally" when the parents become more lax or inconsistent in carrying out the reinforcement program, or the child becomes less interested in the reinforcement. The behavior continues, despite a lack of reinforcement, which now typically is dispensed in a variable ratio format.

Overcorrection.   This disciplinary method incorporates two components: (a) *restitution* and (b) *positive practice*. The former involves correction of damage caused by the misbehavior, while the second involves practicing the desired behavior until it is learned. If an elementary-school aged child has been told repeatedly to pay attention when pouring juice, but he still pours it impulsively and spills juice on the table, restitution will involve cleaning the table, chair, and floor. This would then expand to cleaning an even greater floor area, as well as other chairs. Positive practice would involve repeatedly pouring the juice into a glass with supervision.

A variation of this technique is applicable in the case of the child not wanting to pick up her toys. She can be informed that she has the choice of picking up the toys by herself, or the parent can have her pick the toys up by guiding the child's hands while she is picking up the toys, and also having the child do some additional straightening up of the room.

This approach is quite effective, with the child selecting the "I'll do it myself" option fairly rapidly. If a child is aggressive to another, having the child apologize, give a toy to the child receiving the infraction, or imposing penalties and "fines" are related interventions.

Social Learning Theory/Modeling

The third type of learning is also termed *observational learning, incidental learning, imitation,* or *vicarious learning*. The basic premise is that children learn things merely by watching (Bandura, 1997). There is no apparent reinforcement, and the behavior is simply observed. Some type of cognitive mediation is postulated to occur, and as a result, the learning is considered $S \rightarrow O \rightarrow R$ (stimulus, cognitive operation, response). In day-to-day situations, the child may learn aggressive behavior if a parent frequently displays such; if classmates use foul language, the child may also try it out. If a neighborhood peer whines to get what she wants in front of the child, he might employ that tactic in the future. This phenomenon explains the success of shows such as Sesame Street, or, conversely, the less desirable effects of viewing television violence.

The "classic" example of social learning theory/modeling involved children watching a model engaging in aggressive behavior toward an inflatable Bobo doll (Bandura, Ross, & Ross, 1961). Some children viewed the aggression, while others simple viewed the model in the room with Bobo, but not engaging in any aggressive act. When subsequently placed in a similar situation, those children who witnessed the aggression had a greater likelihood of displaying aggression (two times more likely) than those who did not witness that behavior. In general, modeling increases if the person who is being modeled is reinforced, if the model is held in high regard by the child, if there is perceived similarity between the model and child, and if situations in which the behavior is displayed are similar. This is the basic premise underlying the use of sports stars to endorse various products.

Similarly, modeling can produce an inhibition of behavior. For example, if a child is disruptive and blurts out answers in the classroom, and this results in the teacher firmly reprimanding him in front of the class and imposing restrictions such as loss of recess, the likelihood of classmates disruptively blurting out answers is decreased. It should be emphasized that modeling often occurs in conjunction with other learning paradigms, and in fact, "pure" classical conditioning, respondent conditioning or modeling is not as frequent as one might expect; as elements of each often overlap.

SUMMARY

Although the bulk of this chapter addressed behavioral theories, behavioral techniques should be used in conjunction with consideration of parental, child and developmental concerns. Appreciation of parent issues can produce interventions that are more likely to be accepted and employed. This undoubtedly would enhance compliance. Similarly, appreciating a child's temperament, limitations in cognitive or communication abilities, stage of development, or vulnerable child status, will facilitate development of a more effective and successful intervention. This would also avoid the pitfall of implementation of programs that might be inappropriate for a given child because of unidentified issues or reinforcers. Therefore, a multifaceted, holistic approach is more effective, and affords a greater likelihood of producing change that will persist and be incorporated into day-to-day interactions. The intervention would simply be better tailored to the needs of the child and family and have a higher probability of success. In addition, interventions undertaken in the overall context of a behavioral management program should not underestimate the value of parent education. Subsequent chapters will demonstrate application of this broad-based approach.

Chapter 6

General Intervention Algorithm

It is difficult to employ a "cookbook" method in the treatment of behavioral problems because the child and family each possess unique characteristics. As a result, no one shoe fits all. Nonetheless, a general framework for defining and addressing behavioral problems is useful, with the option of individualized aspects being incorporated in each step. This general algorithm is outlined below and will be referred to throughout this chapter and again throughout Chapter 8.

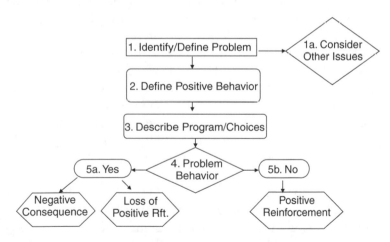

General Intervention Algorithm

IDENTIFY/DEFINE PROBLEM

The practitioner should meet with the parents initially, observe the parent-child interaction, and also see the child individually. Incidental waiting room and hallway vignettes often are highly informative. For example, if the parent constantly asks the child's permission to accompany the clinician for the initial interview, or pleads with the child to remain in the waiting room (e.g., "will you wait here while mommy talks to the doctor?" or "can you play here for a little while?"), this might be indicative of a lack of parental "presence." How the parent(s) handle the child's interruptions (e.g., coming into the room, calling out to them with requests or demands) also provides diagnostic clues regarding the behavioral problem. While the practitioner must be cautious in overgeneralizing, these samples of behavior have a high likelihood of occurring in other situations as well.

When queried regarding the behavioral problem that prompted the visit, parents often have a litany of complaints, and because they want everything to change immediately, they are unfocused and overwhelmed. Stated differently, they are unable to see the trees for the forest. This, in fact, is one of the reasons that parents' attempts to change behavior on their own are unsuccessful; they attempt to address too many things at once, thereby decreasing the likelihood of adequately addressing any single problem. Moreover, they are less likely to be consistent in the institution of any intervention because of the greater number of behaviors to be addressed and the concomitant increased probability of not maintaining a consistent, systematic approach.

A metaphor often presented to parents is they are like an army; however, their troops are constantly involved in skirmishes and as a result, are fatigued and stretched too thinly. As a result, they have no reserve force or adequate concentration of fresh troops to thwart a major offensive thrust mounted by the opposition. However, if the less important firefights could be avoided (i.e., the parents could choose their battles), there would be increased, more concentrated strength available to deal with the more significant, offensive incursion. In other words, parents should ignore unimportant misbehavior, and, at least initially, even misbehavior that is somewhat serious and instead focus efforts on the target behavior that is being addressed.

It is helpful for the parents to develop a list of the three most problematic behaviors. These behaviors must be specific and well defined. For example, "he won't listen," "he has an attitude," or "she's disrespectful" are too vague. Similarly, even a complaint such as "she's aggressive" needs to be broken down into components such as she hits, bites, screams and kicks. These are more concrete examples and can be addressed with specific interventions. This will be important in defining the problem behavior for the child as well (item #3 below). The targeted problem behaviors should have a fairly high rate of occurrence, and produce a significant amount of discomfort for caretakers. The reason for these selection criteria is that parents are more likely to be motivated to change these behaviors, and if the major problems can be successfully handled, the parents will become convinced that this approach really does work and compliance will be enhanced. On the child side, it also provides the implicit message that the parents mean "business."

While a baseline log of the frequency of the problem behavior would be desirable, this tends to be a luxury. Parents understandably want something done as soon as possible. Therefore, when the 3-item problem list is generated, the practitioner needs to determine the duration of the problem, when it occurs (e.g., at dinnertime, early morning, or around the clock), how often it occurs, and in where it is displayed. Evaluating the *pattern* of situations in which the problem behaviors occur may also give clues as to the etiology. Hence, occurrence at home, daycare, school, or in group activities should be determined. If, for example, the problem occurs only at home, this is suggestive of parental permissiveness. While the parents may be dismayed to hear such, in actuality the outcome is more optimistic because the problem behaviors are not pervasive or severe, and there are indications that the child can keep these behaviors in check, if necessary. A caveat is warranted in the school-aged child, however. Some children maintain appropriate behavior in school, despite academic or peer difficulties. However, upon returning home, the stress of the day is discharged, and unfortunately, the parents and other family members bear the brunt of it. If the behavior spills over into other situations, there typically is external pressure on the parents to do something. This may be motivating, or, in some cases, the parents are resentful about this recommendation and may simply be seeing the practitioner to placate others. This issue needs to be explored in more detail, as the ramifications with regard to persistence and passive non-compliance are significant.

Antecedents to the problem behavior need to be identified, as do *consequences*. For example, if a child throws a tantrum every time she is told "no" and the parent simply tells the child that the behavior is "not nice," the antecedents and consequences are readily apparent and amenable to change. It is helpful to gauge the degree of consistency as well. Practitioners should directly question the parent regarding their "consistency percentage"; i.e., is the parent, on average, consistent 50% of the time, 25%, or 75%? It is critical to identify the reinforcers that come into play because these need to be eliminated, and when the behavior is no longer reinforced, the child is faced with an operant extinction situation. This, in conjunction with consequences (5a below) should decrease the frequency of the undesirable behavior. With *functional behavioral analysis* the antecedent (A), behavior (B), and consequence (C) (ABC), as well as the setting and time are identified.

CONSIDER OTHER ISSUES

In addition, several other family-related variables need to be evaluated in the overall assessment of a problem. These include:

- Are both parents in agreement that this behavior is a problem?
- Do both parents use similar disciplinary techniques?
- Are there other family members who have a major role in care-giving and do these individuals see the situation as problematic (e.g., grandparents)?
- What type of environment does the child spend substantial amounts of time in (e.g., a home-based daycare) and what disciplinary methods are routinely employed?
- Do sibling issues have an impact on the current problem?

Developmental issues, temperament, stresses affecting the parents, parenting styles, and attitudes toward misbehavior must be weighed as well. Care must be taken to explore possible stresses that may be directly or indirectly affecting the child.

Finally, child-related issues such as an attention deficit hyperactivity disorder, communication disorder, or learning problems need to be identified and considered in the development of any intervention program. Oftentimes, improving a child's *competencies* in these areas (medi-cation for ADHD, provision of speech-language intervention or learning disabilities assistance) will assist in reducing the problem behavior.

DEFINE POSITIVE BEHAVIOR

As mentioned previously, discipline involves instructing the child as to what to do, as well as what not to do. Therefore, it is very helpful to define positive behaviors that are more desirable and also incompatible with the problem behavior that is being addressed. Essentially, this means strengthening the connection between a positive behavior and reinforcement, while simultaneously emphasizing the ties between misbehavior and negative consequences. It is much more effective to provide the child with an alternative behavior that is reinforced than to simply tell him not to do something and leave it up to him to come up with a more appropriate response. This is particularly necessary when working with younger children. For example, "do not hit your little brother" can be paired with "play nice with him"; "don't run away" and "come to me when I call you"; or "walk, don't run." When the child engages in the more positive, alternative behavior, verbal praise, and tangible reinforcements (the latter administered on a variable ratio schedule) should be dispensed.

DESCRIBE PROGRAM/CHOICES

At the initiation of an intervention, the program needs to be outlined for the child in a simple, concrete, but firm manner. This should occur at a neutral time, and not when emotions are running high. Basically, the problem behavior needs to be clearly delineated and the consequences of a specific action need to be stated in an, "if _____ (specific behavior) occurs then _____ (specific consequence) will happen." It is also important to specify both the desired behavior and the related positive outcome, as well as the negative behavior and its consequence. This is important for several reasons. First, it allows the child to feel in control, although the choices have already been predetermined by the caretaker. It is not unusual for the child to opt for the "wrong" choice on occasion, simply to test the limits of the program and the resolve of the parents—particularly if the behavior had been reinforced previously. Second, this framework provides a learning experience that extends beyond the single behavior being addressed. The child will be developing a life-long behavioral pattern of making choices and then dealing with consequences of those choices. This procedure teaches the child to be responsible for her decisions and the consequences that may follow such decisions.

There also should be no debate as to whether the rule has been broken or not. Once the behaviors are specified, the parent has the authority to decide if the problem behavior was emitted. Arguing or debating the infraction simply gets the parent sidetracked and raises the possibility that the child might inadvertently be reinforced for the problem behavior, or at least derive some satisfaction that he has irritated the parent during the course of the protest.

PROBLEM BEHAVIOR

The problem behavior must be defined specifically; if it occurs, even in a mild form (e.g., the tantrum was very brief), it should be followed by the predetermined consequence. It is not unusual for parents to allow less intense variants of the problem behavior slide. Basically, the parents' infraction threshold varies, depending on their interpretation of the severity and intent of the problem behavior. However, this confuses the child, and tends to raise the possibility of inconsistency. Therefore, during the initial intervention, it is better to be a bit more liberal in dispensing consequences than allowing an infraction to occur without a consequence. Stated differently, at this stage it is best to interpret the behavior in a yes/no versus a "shades of gray" manner.

IF PROBLEM BEHAVIOR OCCURS

If the problem behavior occurs, it must be consistently followed by a consequence. The two most effective techniques to use with young children are *time outs* and *response cost*. These can be used individually or in tandem.

Time Out

Time out from positive reinforcement is probably the most common form of discipline. This technique refers to the orchestrated removal of positive reinforcers for a specified period of time following the occurrence of undesirable behavior. Stated differently, time out refers to removal from "time in" (Parrish, 1999). There are two types of time out: (1) *exclusionary* time out, and (2) *non-exclusionary* time out. The former involves the child being sent to his room, a corner, or a chair situated in a quiet place. Essentially, the child is removed from so-called "time-in" (reinforcement). With non-exclusionary time out, the child remains in the situation, but cannot engage in the desired act for a specified amount of time. Here, the reinforcement is removed from the child, and this is equivalent to the aforementioned response cost.

For example, assume a child will not stop playing a videogame on the television in the family room, despite the warning that if he did not stop, he would receive a time out. Exclusionary time out would involve removing the child from the family room to a time out area, and having him remain in a seat for a specified amount of time. In non-exclusionary time out (response cost), the videogame controls would be taken away from the child for the rest of the evening, even though he might still stay in the family room. A more stringent variant or combination, would be to use both types in tandem, namely send the child out of the room for a time out, and also prohibit playing videogames for the rest of the evening.

Generally, exclusionary time out is most effective in the 2- to 6- or 7-year age range, and is best applied to tantrums, aggression, noncompliance or other negative behaviors. It should not be applied to avoidance, escape, or fear-related behaviors. Grounding is an example of time-out applied to older children and adolescents.

Time-Out Enhancement

There are several suggestions that enhance the effectiveness of exclusionary time out. These are:

- Time out should be immediate and initially applied only to targeted behaviors.

- If possible, time out should be administered in a consistent place, that is out of the mainstream of family activity.
- Time out should be preceded by a single warning (if it is in response to aggression such as hitting a parent, no warnings should be given).
- It should be of a predetermined duration (the popular rule of thumb is one minute per year of age, however this seems to be more for mnemonic purposes than based on science. This also would not be appropriate for children of older ages). Nonetheless, it is useful for parents to follow this guideline for preschoolers and early school-age children.
- Young children (<5 years) should not be placed in time out for longer than 10 minutes; if a younger child remains in time out too long, she often forgets why she was placed there in the first place.
- With young children, if they cry, whine or fidget in the time out chair, they do not need to remain in time out until they are quiet or still. Doing so would simply divert the focus to being quiet, versus why the child was placed in time out to begin with (thereby reducing its efficacy). However, if the child becomes verbally abusive to the parent while in time out, extending time and adding response costs are definite options.
- With older children (e.g., >5 or 6 years of age), a prerequisite for ending time out could be that the child must now be quiet.
- A timer is helpful; it is concrete, allows the child to grasp the concept, and avoids the child incessantly asking the parent if time is up yet (which would provide interaction and negate the "exclusionary" component).
- There should be no verbal exchanges while the child is in time out.
- Similarly, yelling nagging, threatening or being verbally demeaning should be avoided when attempting to institute time out. If the child refuses to go, "physical guidance" should be employed.
- If a child refuses to stay in time out, several options are available. First a "step-up" procedure could be employed, whereby if the child refuses stay in the time-out chair, she will be warned that the next step is her room. If she continues to be non-compliant, then she should be placed in her room with the door open. If she insists on coming out of the room, then the door should be shut (and held by the parent—not locked). In such cases, all toys and "fun" things should be removed from the room prior to using it for time out. Some children become destructive when placed in their room for time out. If a child kicks the door, remove his shoes; if he throws objects, remove them; if he empties dresser drawers and messes up the room, overcorrection should be employed.

- If a child occasionally leaves the time out chair, he should be escorted back and some time added for the infraction (resetting the entire time often is not productive, particularly for younger children).
- At the culmination of time out, the child should be told by the parent in a matter-of-fact manner what the problem behavior was, and what a more appropriate behavior would have been. A warning should also be delivered to the child, indicating that similar behavior would not be tolerated and would result in yet another time out.
- Restraining a child by holding her in time out often is not effective because the child is reinforced for the problem behavior (attention), and many children slam their heads backward, struggle the entire time, or make the situation so unbearable for the parents that they may tend to shy away from implementation of the intervention.
- Rather than repeatedly increasing the duration of time out because the child is being non-compliant, it may be better to fold in additional response costs (e.g., loss of television, going out to play, computer time) in an incremental fashion.

As stated previously, time out is more effective if positive reinforcement is also provided for more appropriate behavior. In addition, the impact of time out is enhanced if the child is then allowed to once again enter the same situation (so-called time in) and now engages in a more acceptable behavior (e.g., playing nicely with sibling, versus hitting her). Problems that may detract from the effectiveness of time-out will be discussed in the next chapter.

Response Cost

Response cost involves withdrawal of a privilege or imposition of a penalty. In the former, if the child repeatedly leaves the yard when she has been warned not to do so, being allowed to go in the yard by herself is now stopped. An additional penalty would involve the child going to the door and telling her friends she has to stay in the rest of the day, and also part of tomorrow as well. Response cost is most effective if the child greatly values the reinforcer. Practitioners will often hear parents say imposition of response cost does not "bother" the child; this simply means they haven't selected something that the child really wants to have or do. Similarly, if the child tells the parents that he doesn't care about the consequence, this does not necessarily mean it has no effect on him.

Parents need to realize that the child is certainly not going admit that a consequence is really getting to him; moreover, there might be the underlying hope that by saying that the consequence is ineffective, the parents might desist in implementation of that particular punishment.

IF PROBLEM BEHAVIOR DOES NOT OCCUR

If the problem behavior does not occur, it is advisable to provide both a short-term and a long-term reinforcement, with specific praise being directed to the desirable behavior that was displayed. The use of both types of reinforcement is necessary because young children do not have the cognitive capacity for long delays, and therefore are not as motivated by the possibility of reinforcement being delivered after several days or weeks of appropriate behavior. For example, telling a child that she will receive a bike after a month of consecutive days in which she did not receive a circle for misbehavior in her kindergarten classroom: (a) would almost be impossible to achieve; and (b) would not have any intermediary reinforcement that would sustain the behavior long-term. Long-term reinforcement is more effective if it is based on cumulative, versus consecutive, days. Conversely, providing only short-term rewards may or may not be as effective as also offering a more cumulative reinforcer that would encourage more sustained, goal-directed behavior. An example of the combined use of a short and long-term reinforcement would be to have the child be able to go into a "grab-bag" or "treasure chest" upon completion of a day without the non-desired behavior (e.g., temper tantrum). In addition to the privilege of going into the grab-bag, the child also receives a sticker on a calendar. Once a specified number of stickers have been acquired (e.g., 4, not necessarily in a row, but rather, as mentioned previously, acquired cumulatively) then the child can have a more substantial reward, such as a trip to a fast-food restaurant, a special trip to the museum, a movie, or renting a videotape.

This intervention algorithm can be applied to most behavioral problems in young children with components being individually selected for specific situations (in terms of target behaviors, reinforcers and consequences). Fine-tuning is typically necessary, but this procedure actually is diagnostic in and of itself, as it provides the clinician with information on parental behaviors and persistence, as well as that of the child. More specific intervention components are found in the following chapter.

Chapter 7

Specific Techniques

There exist a variety of techniques that can be applied to address behavioral problems. Some are more useful than others, and in an effort to assist the practitioner, these techniques are rated on a five-star format, with more desirable approaches receiving more stars. Whenever any technique is employed, the practitioner must be certain to request that the caretaker recount exactly what has been implemented, so as to fine tune the program, and correct any misconceptions or less-than-optimal applications.

STATEMENTS OF DISAPPROVAL/EXPLANATIONS (***)

Verbal responses may consist of warnings, threats, reprimands, or explanations. In general the behavioral effects of these techniques are variable and inconsistent at best. As a result, these are given a three-star rating *if used in isolation*. One issue that influences efficacy is the frequency of use. While such responses often take on the role of a negative reinforcer, excessive use tends to vitiate efficacy, with the child becoming immune or accustomed to reprimands or explanations. Stated differently, the child simply becomes habituated and tunes these statements out. Conversely, if applied judiciously, a reprimand can serve as a cue that the behavior is significantly out of line.

Occasionally, statements of disapproval may provide negative attention, thereby actually becoming reinforcing. The mode of delivery is important as well; reprimands often are given in the midst of a high level of emotion. This can serve to misdirect the intervention away from the actual infraction, because emotions override any learning. Caretakers must be careful to not directly attack a child's self esteem; if criticism is delivered, it must be in relation to the behavior and not the child. Making a statement such as "you're a good kid, but what you did was wrong," or "you made a bad choice," is appropriate. A terse (versus long-winded) explanation of the behavior and consequence and a personalized reference such as, "I don't like that," are helpful as well. Statements of disapproval are not effective consequences in and of themselves. They are much more effective if used in conjunction with other methods.

Warnings

Warnings are only effective if they are followed by action. Similarly, threats typically involve emotions and often are delivered several times before a consequence is employed—therefore both of these techniques actually cause the parent to become even more inconsistent and would tend to maintain, and not eliminate, the problem behavior. Therefore, verbal techniques can be more effective if:

- The parent has "presence" or established credibility that he/she will indeed implement a stated consequence.
- Such reprimands, statements of disapproval or warnings are doled out judiciously.
- They are delivered in a firm, but not emotional manner.
- The child's self-esteem and self-concept are not attacked.
- The vignette does not deteriorate into an argument or shouting match.
- The verbal approach is not used as the solitary intervention.
- The explanation is not long and complicated.
- The child is not placed in control with statements such as, "you hurt mommy's feelings."

Conversely, *verbal approval* is a potent reinforcer, particularly if the parent-child relationship is strong. It can readily be used as an alternative to verbal disapproval, and if employed wisely, simple withdrawal of verbal approval may become a very effective technique as well.

A cautionary note regarding verbal threats is warranted. Threats are typically ineffective because they are not followed by prompt action. They often are vague or unclear, and they are dispensed inconsistently. Threats often are a sign of parental desperation, as evident by the yelling and often unreasonable consequences that are voiced (e.g., "you'll never watch television again!").

TIME OUT (*****)

Time out was discussed in Chapter 6. Exclusionary time out is probably the most common and effective intervention with toddlers and young children, the age range of efficacy ranging from 2 years up to age 6 or 7. It may be used with children who are a few years older, and perhaps even down to 18-months, but the effects are diminished. Time out involves removal of the child from reinforcement because of an undesirable behavior (or "time-in"; Parrish, 1999). This technique is best applied to more negative, externalizing behaviors. The preferred time-out location is a chair that is out of the mainstream of family activity. Parents should also have a strategy in place for time-out escape or non-compliance. As mentioned earlier, a step-up procedure can be employed whereby if the child does not sit in the chair or runs away, the next scenario would be to place the child in his room with the door open. If he repeatedly comes out, then the door should be closed (and held closed, not locked). If the child is destructive, then environmental engineering must be employed ahead of time to prevent damage or injury. Continued escalation should be met with addition of other "costs," versus continuously adding additional time to the procedure. If escalation occurs, the parents' behavioral repertoire in response to the escalation is restricted if the addition of more penalty time is the only alternative; therefore, adding loss of privileges, overcorrection, or other techniques is preferred.

To reiterate an earlier point, this author does not recommend restraining (holding) a noncompliant child until she calms down. This isn't truly a time out, as the child receives much attention, the conflict could extend well beyond the recommended time-out duration. Moreover, the focus shifts from the child making a connection between the infraction and consequence, to the fear involved in a show of physical force. Furthermore, there is a possibility that the parent may be injured by a misdirected head-butt to the nose, or even more intentional aggression. As a result, parents will be less inclined to implement this technique, with a resultant increase in inconsistency.

Time out should be preceded by *one warning* and if the undesirable behavior persists, then time out is implemented as soon as possible. If too many warnings are given, the warning again loses its value as a cue, and the first several will have no impact. A statement of disapproval can be delivered as well. Techniques that enhance the efficacy of time out are delineated in Chapter 6.

If Time Out is Ineffective

If time out is ineffective, there are several considerations that should be evaluated. These include:

- The time out is either too short or too long in duration.
- Confusion exists regarding what behavior specifically warrants time out.
- An argument ensues.
- The child receives negative attention from time out.
- No warning or cue is provided by the parent.

- Time out is applied inconsistently.
- Time out is over-applied to numerous situations in an indiscrimi-nant fashion (i.e., it is used excessively).
- It is not administered in a timely fashion (although delay between infraction and time out can be longer with older children).
- Time-out is preferred by the child to avoid engaging in a more undesired behavior (such as cleaning one's room). In such cases, the time out is delivered for the refusal, and then the child is allowed to have another chance to carry out the original request. Continued refusal would then warrant another time out.
- The child is too young (<18 months) or too old (where a reason-able duration of time-out would not be effective).
- People continue to interact with the child while he is in time-out.

Time out provides structure for the child with a predictable, behavior → consequence chain. As mentioned previously, while a child might com-plain about such structure, in actuality, structure is reassuring for the child and provides a sense of security. It also enhances learning and hones the child's decision-making abilities.

PRESENTATION OF AVERSIVE STIMULI (*)

Aversive stimuli that are presented contingent upon the child demons-trating an undesirable behavior include spanking, placing soap in the child's mouth, squirting the youngster with a water bottle, frightening the child (by turning all the lights out in her room), or mandating that the child engage in the non-desired behavior repeatedly, are not recommended. These techniques are intrusive, and, in some cases, border on being abu-sive. They are not effective and may cause the child to suppress the behav-ior only in a specific situation, thereby becoming more covert or secretive as well. Modeling occurs and the child learns that dominance is achieved by force. The intensity of the aversive stimuli again disrupts the learning association, with the child attempting to avoid the consequence and not considering the infraction. Suffice it to say that it is not advisable for the practitioner to recommend such behavioral interventions to parents.

RESPONSE COST (*****)

This technique may also be considered non-exclusionary time-out because the reinforcement is taken away from the child (versus the child being removed from the reinforcing situation). This involves a positive reinforcement being taken away or a penalty (negative consequence) imposed. Typically, the child loses a privilege or access to a reinforcing object. Response cost is most effective if the consequence can be directly related to the infraction, this being termed logical consequences. For example, if a child were destructive with a toy, then the response cost, delivered after one warning, would be loss of the use of that toy for a specified amount of time. One pitfall that parents sometimes encounter in the application of response cost is failure to realize that the response cost must also have, as a necessary component, the possibility of regaining the desired object. Therefore, telling the child that the toy will be put in the trash or that she will not be able to watch television for a month is not effective. The loss must be realistic and something that can be implemented and followed through on. If not, then the risk of inconsistency is increased dramatically. Care must be taken to identify privileges or objects that the child truly desires. Increased satiation lessens the impact of the loss; deprivation enhances the salience of the intervention. Therefore, response cost is most effective if:

- The consequence is specified clearly and the duration of the penalty is realistic and can be implemented (if it is outrageous, the child will not perceive it as being credible).
- There is an opportunity to regain the privilege or object once the penalty has been implemented.
- The consequence is related to the infraction (e.g., excessive use of a video game would result in loss of that privilege for the rest of the day).
- The consequence is amenable to a step-up procedure.
- The desirability of the privilege or object is high and satiation does not exist.
- Logical or natural consequences are employed.

Conversely, if application of response cost is not effective, then the practitioner should consider the following:

- There has been a variable or inconsistent application of consequences.
- The child simply did not care about the loss of the object or privilege, the parent realizing that any child is not likely to tell the parent that he is bothered by a consequence.
- The parent routinely does not follow-through for the specified amount of time the child will not have the object or engage in an activity.
- There are too many other activities or objects that can replace the one lost to the penalty.

- The initial consequence is such that the ability for subsequent step-up is precluded.
- It is better for a response cost to be of a lesser intensity or magnitude, but have a more realistic probability of being implemented, than to threaten a severe penalty, but not follow through.

TOKEN SYSTEMS (*****)

This intervention strategy involves giving chips, stars, checks, coupons, stickers, or tickets, contingent upon demonstration of a desired behavior, or inhibition of a non-desirable behavior. These items are secondary reinforcers and therefore have to be tied into a more tangible, primary reinforcement. More specifically, chips, coupons, stickers, or stars lose their reinforcing value if they are not redeemed for something that is more desired. Pragmatically, these techniques are best if they have both a short and long term component. For example, a sticker can be placed on a calendar and the child would be allowed to go into a "grab-bag" or "treasure chest" (described subsequently) at the end of the day. Accumulation of a specified number of stickers would then afford the child the opportunity for a larger reward. Such programs should not be overly elaborate, as this tends to confuse the child, particularly at younger ages. It is helpful to develop reward menus in which the child has the option of selecting different rewards for a prerequisite number of accumulated stickers, or if coupons are used, a graduated reward menu can be developed in which more expensive or desirable rewards require greater expenditure of coupons.

Token programs can be used: (a) to increase the likelihood of a behavior that otherwise would have a low probability of occurring; or (b) as an adjunct reinforcer for cessation of a problem behavior such as aggression, used in conjunction with a technique such as time out for the occurrence of the non-desirable behavior.

Token programs need to be explained to the child beforehand. It is also beneficial to employ social or activity rewards with family members as the long-term component. This approach would be particularly powerful if, during the course of the definition of the problem, it was determined that the child is highly desirous of attention, or there is a great deal of sibling rivalry. Such one-on-one time for the parent and child would be highly reinforcing to the child and also would provide incentive for more prosocial behavior. Even if the desire for parental contact is not a driving force, this activity provides quality time and would enhance the parent-child relationship. Bonus tokens or stickers can be given for exceptionally good behavior, thereby further enhancing the likelihood of the desired behavior. Changes in the reward menu tend to maintain the child's interest, just as revamping of restaurant menus pleases regular clientele.

GRAB-BAG/TREASURE CHEST (*****)

This technique consists of a short-term reinforcement in which a child, after a day of not displaying a problem behavior or after receiving a specified number of stars for demonstration of appropriate behavior, is allowed to go into a grocery bag, box, or similar container, to retrieve a prize. The grab-bag should include inexpensive items such as matchbox cars, toy figures, writing instruments, doll accessories, collectible cards, food treats, bead bracelets, toy jewelry or other objects that are desirable to the child. Children involved in this procedure should participate in selection of the items, and it should be verified that these items have reinforcement value. The program should be made "easier" initially (vis à vis *shaping*), so as to encourage the child and have him experience success and a reinforcement.

For example, if a child with a toileting problem receives one sticker each time she sits on the toilet, and two stickers if there is an actual bowel movement, it would be advisable to start the program with the requirement that two stickers qualify for a trip to the grab-bag. This requirement for reinforcement could subsequently be increased to three stickers, then four stickers, and so on. Conversely, once the program has been established and the desired behavior is frequent, a fading procedure can be employed, whereby the child receives stickers only for having a bowel movement, or the number of stickers necessary for a reinforcement increases. Fading often occurs naturally, with the child being less reward-dependent or enthusiastic, yet the desired behavior is maintained. During the course of a grab-bag intervention, the items contained in the grab-bag should be varied, so as to maintain the child's interest.

There exist many variations to this procedure. Use of a box or chest (hence, the name, "treasure chest") instead of a bag is one such modification. Some parents have used five shoeboxes with different numbers, colors, or pictures on each box; the child then earns a random coupon with one of the corresponding numbers, colors or pictures, and is allowed to obtain the prize in that particular shoebox. This technique is labor-intensive, but does maintain the child's interest and adds another dimension of excitement. Yet another variation involves the child starting with a certain number of coupons or tokens, with loss of the reinforcers incurred when the undesirable behavior is displayed, in so doing depleting the amount that was initially awarded to the child. Again, a reward menu for redeeming the coupons or tokens must be developed. The ability to earn back tokens for appropriate behavior also is useful. Token programs can be enhanced by sibling competitiveness. It sometimes is helpful to have siblings of the identified patient also placed on a token program for some other behavior that is a subthreshold problem. Rewards take on a new dimension if one sibling receives a reinforcement and the other does not. Token programs are more effective if they are tied in to long-term rewards as well.

If Token Program is Unsuccessful

If the token or sticker program does not work, parents and practitioners should consider the following possibilities:

- The procedure is too confusing or complex for the child to understand.
- The program initially is not restricted to one behavior, and therefore is over-applied.
- Because of excessively stringent criteria, the child does not have the opportunity to experience success and a reward.
- The shaping procedure moves ahead too quickly.
- Rewards are not dispensed properly (i.e., the parent forgets).
- Items are not reinforcing to the child, and he habituates to the program.
- The child has an opportunity for misbehavior after the reinforcement has been given too early in the day (e.g., immediately after dinner, thereby leaving several hours for potential misbehavior afterward, versus allowing access to the grab-bag later in the evening).
- The fading procedure was implemented too quickly, typically before the desired behavior has become strong.
- "Secondary reinforcers" such as stickers, stars, or tickets, are not tied in to a more tangible reinforcement (grab-bag, treasure chest).
- The program is punctuated by use of corporal punishment, yelling, or berating the child.

IGNORING/DISTRACTING (***)

As mentioned previously in the discussion of extinction, ignoring can be useful under certain circumstances. Ignoring is particularly applicable for temper tantrums or whining/crying that occurs with little provocation.

Parents need to exercise caution when ignoring a child's behavior, as in some cases they may unknowingly reinforce the misbehavior by "ignoring" it, when in actuality, the child is cognizant of the fact that the behavior is annoying the parent (even though the parent tries to provide the impression that it does not work). In such situations, behaviors that the child emits may have a reinforcing value in and of themselves and ignoring the behavior without a concomitant consequence or penalty would not be effective. Obviously, ignoring a behavior that is directly reinforcing to the child is not effective. Therefore, situations in which ignoring might be useful include:

- When the parent is implementing a new intervention, and needs to focus on a more specific, relevant behavior (thereby ignoring other, less important behaviors at that point).
- If it is determined that attention is a major reinforcer, even if it is negative attention.
- The problem behavior is low-intensity.
- The child or others are not in danger, and there is no destructive behavior.
- If ignoring is paired with a consequence or "cost" for the misbehavior (such as time-out or loss of privilege).

Related to ignoring is the technique of *distracting*. This technique is most effective in younger children, and basically involves the parent derailing a problem before it develops too much intensity. For example, if a youngster is reluctant to give up a toy during a testing session, it is much more appropriate for the examiner to distract his attention with a different toy than to engage in a tug-of-war with him to wrestle away the original one. This approach is particularly useful in sidestepping tantrums, or in preventing the child from taking a stand on a trivial issue, due to the need to establish autonomy. Distracting is best applied in low-intensity situations, and should be viewed as a preventative, versus remedial measure.

BEHAVIOR LOG/DIARY (*****)

A behavior log or diary provides clues to the parents regarding a given behavioral problem. It helps them focus on a specific behavior, and the record provides quantitative data regarding a baseline and improvement in behavior. It also enables parents to monitor their own behaviors more systematically. Similarly, the log enables the practitioner to detect patterns in behaviors that can then guide interventions. A calendar with stars or stickers is useful for this purpose, however it would only show those occasions or days when the child received reinforcement, and would not provide information about the number or type of infractions, antecedents, or consequences. Nonetheless, calendars are a powerful tool to demonstrate to the child how successful she is.

With a log or diary, it is helpful to have: (1) time of day that the problem behavior occurred, (2) antecedent behavior (child *and* parent), (3) specific type of infraction (what it was, level of intensity), (4) consequence for the infraction, and (5) child's reaction to the disciplinary technique (acceptance, anger, yelling). This is along the lines of the ABC (antecedent, behavior, consequence) procedure mentioned earlier, but is a bit more detailed. Practitioners must inform the parents about the typical intensification or "burst" of problem behaviors that often occurs with initiation of a given intervention, again emphasizing that paradoxically, this increase is indicative of the effectiveness of the intervention because of the magnitude of the child's protests (what was paying off no longer is, and the child finds that very distressing). In so doing, the parents will not be as dismayed by the initial, apparent ineffectiveness of the intervention or be deterred by the intensification of problem behaviors. Careful review of the log by the practitioner will provide clues regarding patterns of behavior, and pinpoint where intervention may benefit from fine-tuning.

A simple example involves reviewing a log and noting a recurrent pattern in which a child throws temper tantrums when told "no." If the consequence is a verbal reprimand, there is an eventual reduction in the intensity of the tantrum, but afterwards, there are multiple recurrences in a relatively short amount of time. This is contrast to situations noted in the log where the temper tantrums are immediately followed by a time-out, which again leads to a reduction in behavior. However, under these circumstances, there are fewer later recurrences. By reviewing the log, it becomes clear to the practitioner and demonstrates to the parents that certain interventions (time-outs) will have a greater impact than others (reprimands) on preventing recurrence of the problem behaviors later on. This pattern might not have been detected with sole use of a calendar with stickers.

Parents should not "forget" to bring the log to follow-up appointments. When this occurs, the possibility of non-compliance in administration of the program is raised, because if the parents cannot systematically complete a log, they most likely cannot muster the effort needed to implement behavioral change. With respect to the calendar, it is very useful to have the child bring it affixed with the appropriate stickers to the follow-up appointment in order to show the practitioner and receive praise and encouragement.

OTHER APPROACHES/CONSIDERATIONS (*****)

Perhaps the most important, yet most elusive factor in behavioral management is the parents' "discipline mindset." More specifically, this involves several questions: (a) do the parents see the behavior as problematic? (b) are they willing to do something about it? (c) are *both* parents in agreement regarding the magnitude of the problem and the need to address it? and (d) do they believe the intervention will work? An affirmative answer to all four questions is necessary, but the last question is the most critical, and the one most likely to not be endorsed wholeheartedly. After all, the parents understandably often believe that they have adequately attempted to change things, but to no avail. Therefore, they are skeptical that a new, relatively simple program would be more successful than what has already been tried. The message that parents *must* convey to the child is that they are serious, determined, and "mean it" when they are addressing the problem behavior. This attitude of assuredness transmits to the child the message that this intervention *will* work, thereby altering the child's expectations as well. If the parent(s) has doubts and expresses ambivalence, this cue is readily detected by the child and decreases the likelihood of success. Parental emotions need to be excluded from the mix, as this only adds more potential problems. Interventions should be explained ahead of time, in a firm, measured, and reassuring manner. This transmits parental expectation of appropriate behavior to the child in an unthreatening way. This positive expectation and explanation will, in turn, alter the child's attitude as well.

Along these lines, any rules that are employed must be fair, and realistically attainable by the child. Parents should avoid "power struggle" situations where escalation on both sides of the equation is inevitable (Schmitt, 1991). For example, if a child wets his pants purposefully, punishing the child with a spanking for doing so will only exacerbate the behavior. In such cases, withdrawing from the punishment mode, but still having the child be responsible for washing, changing, and cleaning up the area (overcorrection), coupled with positive reinforcement for not wetting, is more desirable.

As mentioned previously, some parents view reinforcing a desired behavior as "*bribery*." Rather than use this term, which has negative connotations and suggests that the parents are simply trying to placate the child, it is better to consider this as an "*incentive*" or "*reinforcement for positive behavior*." Essentially, the caretaker is attempting to shape a new behavior, and this is the means of doing so. Once the behavior is established, the so-called bribery can be faded out. It is helpful to point out to parents that salaries or bonuses for adults serve the same purposes, but are not bribes, per se—they are reinforcements that are delivered upon completion of a task or demonstration of desirable behavior.

With reference to the "discipline mindset," parents should not second guess themselves. If they make a decision, they should stick to it. This argues for planfulness and not reacting emotionally to a situation, if at all possible. Again, ambivalence regarding the "correctness" of the parents' response only serves to detract from the efficacy of the intervention. That is not to say that behavioral interventions should not be reviewed or discussed by parents subsequently; doing so will fine tune the response or provide alternate methods for dealing with similar situations in the future. If the parent conveys self-assuredness, the child will feel more secure as well. Embedded in the mindset is the message that institution of discipline means that the parent cares and it is not counter to nurturance. Parents, in some respects, can also directly influence the immediate future, in that they inform the child (with one warning) that if the behavior does not stop, a specified consequence will follow. While the child controls the choice, the parent controls the subsequent consequences.

In this undertaking, humor is an ally and can often defuse situations by allowing the parent to step back a bit. Humor should be employed whenever possible because:

- It allows both the child and the parent to save face.
- In some cases it reduces the seriousness, and may underscore the triviality, of the incident.
- Humor allows avoidance of unnecessary confrontation and escalation.
- It conveys positive affect, versus anger.
- Humor potentially can expand the child's behavioral repertoire so that she might include humor in adapting to future situations.

As suggested earlier, when delivering a disciplinary message, the parent should use "I" versus "you" (referring to the child). More specifically, saying, "I don't like that behavior," is preferred over "You did a bad thing again." The former method produces less defensiveness on the part of the child, and enhances the likelihood of compliance. Oftentimes, as soon as the child perceives that the situation is one of confrontation, he shuts down and is not receptive to anything that even remotely resembles criticism.

The potent influence of modeling should also not be overlooked. When the parent employs yelling, the child yells back; an aggressive adult produces aggression in the child, while degrading comments directed at the child produce reciprocal anger and verbal hostility (as well as a negative impact on the child's self-esteem). Conversely, measured responding on the part of the parent provides a model for more appropriate, better modulated responses in the child.

Use of maturity-related comments such as being a "big boy" or a "big girl" with young children is often helpful, particularly if the child is in the process of a developmental transition (e.g., moving to a "big girl" bed when graduating from the crib; using "big boy" pants during the transition from pull-ups to underwear).

APPLICATIONS

Throughout the behavioral intervention, the practitioner acts in the role of a coach, doing so non-judgmentally. With this approach, parents are less offended by the clinician critiquing parental behaviors that may contribute to maintaining the problem. Being empathic with questions such as, "How bad does it get?" or "What works to improve the behavior?" is also helpful. This role also attributes success to the parents' efforts and not to the practitioner, although the *burden* of success then is intuitively placed on the parents. Although this might seem to be a ploy on the part of the practitioner to avoid responsibility, in actuality the professional has no control over what happens once the child and her caretaker(s) leave the office, with compliance being totally dependent on the parents.

Therefore, it is incumbent on the practitioner to convey the attitude that the intervention will produce improvement if it is carried out, and modified if necessary. Realistic expectations also should be provided and these include: (1) All children demonstrate some problem behaviors over the course of a given day, (2) Rarely does a behavior totally cease, nor does a desired behavior occur 100% of the time, and (3) The goal is to reduce the problem behavior and increase the desired behavior to an acceptable level that is less stressful and more comfortable for both the child and the parent. Similarly, no parent responds correctly or does the right thing every time a problem behavior occurs. On any given day, fatigue, job stress, time pressures, physical malaise, or the child having a particularly bad day, may cause the parent to react more emotionally, or be less realistic and understanding, or more inconsistent. The key is to be as consistent as possible, so as to avoid emergence of a variable ratio reinforcement schedule (a.k.a., inconsistency, which is highly resistant to extinction). Children are resilient, and a few, minor "mistakes" on the part of the parent should not derail development to an appreciable degree. Parents should be reassured of that fact *specifically*.

A final suggestion regards the concept of "physical presence" or "manual guidance" (Schmitt, 1991). Situations often deteriorate when the parent loses patience because of repeated verbal directives that are not followed. Rather than repeatedly telling the child to do something, and, in the process, becoming increasingly frustrated and angry, it often behooves the parent to physically move to the child's vicinity and direct the behavior. For example, if the child is sent upstairs to go to bed but dawdles, makes multiple excuses, does not turn the light out in the room, or plays, repeatedly yelling upstairs to the child to stop these behaviors would be ineffective. Instead, the parent would be better advised to go upstairs, escort the child to his bed, give hugs and kisses, turn off the light, and provide the directive that the bedtime ritual has now ended. While this does not seem to involve more effort on the front end, in actuality, it probably decreases effort and angst in the long run. This is especially true if the motivation for the child's behavior is stalling or attention-seeking. This approach also is effective in other situations such as when the child is sent to clean her room.

In the following sections, principles and techniques discussed previously will be applied to cases for illustrative purposes.

Chapter 8

Applications

In the next sections, specific problems will be presented to demonstrate application of the concepts discussed previously. These will be addressed via use of the General Intervention Algorithm outlined in Chapter 6. These cases are representative of the broad array of behavioral problems frequently encountered in primary care and underscore the fact that each situation has common elements in addition to unique aspects. Conceptualization of the problem and selection of intervention strategies will also draw on the premises underscored in the *DSM-PC*. It is acknowledged that there often are alternative intervention strategies that might be employed to effectively address these same problems. Moreover, practitioners and parents often devise variations that are unique and innovative.

In general, *problems of daily routines* (see Chapter 1) such as food refusal, bedtime problems, or toileting are most effectively handled with shaping, positive reinforcement, and natural consequences; punishment generally is not effective. With *aggressive-resistant behavior* (negativism, argumentativeness, temper tantrums, aggressiveness), time-outs, response cost, extinction, and positive reinforcement for desired behaviors are the most useful techniques. Providing one warning for the child is appropriate for resistant behaviors, while no warning should be given for physical aggression. In the case of *overdependent/withdrawing behavior* (clinging, whining, refusal to separate), firm limit setting with reassurance, shaping, modeling, and reinforcement for positive behaviors is recommended. *Undesirable habits* such as night awakening, thumbsucking, or excessive masturbation are best reduced by reinforcement of competing behaviors, extinction (ignoring), or, in some cases, shaping.

In applying the concepts and principles outlined in previous sections, the practitioner must appreciate the quandary faced by parents whose child has an identified developmental, physical, or sensory disorder, in conjunction with a behavioral problem. For example, take the case of a child identified as having a sensory integration problem, who is overly stimulated by crowds, resulting in temper tantrums and out-of-control behavior. Parents might be confused when trying to determine whether the temper display is volitional or due to the sensory integration problem. If they attribute the cause for the temper tantrum to sensory overload, they might be more tolerant or permissive regarding the problematic behavior and discount any volitional component. This could also lead to parental indecisiveness that potentially may further exacerbate the tantrums. This scenario can often occur in the presence of other child characteristics such as an attention deficit hyperactivity disorder or an anxiety problem.

While there most likely is an association between the identified disorder and the behavioral problem, this simply means that there is an increased propensity for the behavior because of issues such as the sensory overload, impulsivity in the case of ADHD, or fear in the child with anxiety. Although it is virtually impossible to separate the disorder from the more volitional behavioral component, it is reasonable to inform the parents that although the identified disorder does heighten the probability of the child displaying a problem, (and in all likelihood has contributed to initiation of the problem), how the parents address the behaviors will determine whether they continue, and to what degree. This situation is best conceptualized as consisting of two overlapping circles: the first is the behavioral component, while the second is the identified disorder. The area of overlap between the two circles, namely the behavioral problem, reflects the association between the two.

The area of overlap varies, depending first on the child's propensity for sensory overload, anxiety, or impulsivity. However, more important is the fact that the identified disorder provides the impetus, but the width of the overlapping area (i.e., the behavioral problem) will be affected by how the environment responds to the child's behavior. Caring parents want to prevent discomfort for their child and therefore may tend to attribute the problem behaviors to the identified disorder, and not the child. The situation becomes more complex if the parent had a similar physical, developmental, or neurodevelopmental problem during his or her own childhood.

Hence there are two factors that will determine the area of overlap, and it is often difficult for both the practitioner and the parents to determine the relative contribution of child and environmental characteristics contributing to the behavioral problem.

CASE 1. AGGRESSION

Natalie is a 3-year, 4-month old preschooler who is brought in because of behavioral problems. Her single mom reports that *"nothing makes her (Natalie) happy," and "I can't take her anywhere to have a good time." Natalie also is highly aggressive toward her 6-year-old sister and $1\frac{1}{2}$-year-old brother. Temper tantrums result whenever Natalie is reprimanded or her wants are unmet, and she recently has begun to wet her pants when she becomes angry, both at home and at daycare.*

Identify/Define Problem Generation of the top 3 problem behaviors resulted in the following: (1) hitting and kicking siblings and mother; (2) crying when the mother left Natalie at daycare; and (3) wetting her pants. When asked what type of *consequence* typically followed aggression, the mother indicated that she let Natalie "throw her fit" and then would hold her to calm her down and explain to her why she should not hit people. The impact of the intervention was further diluted by the fact that the mother admittedly intervened sporadically (i.e., <50% of the time). The mother also acknowledged that she typically was tired when she got home from work, and that she sometimes "let things go" rather than have to engage in a confrontation. The problem behavior also surfaces in daycare, and when Natalie becomes aggressive there, her mother is called to take her home. Observation of the mother and child in the examination room revealed the youngster whining, climbing on the mother, and literally getting in the mother's face. In addition, she refused the examiner's requests, and, subsequently, launched into temper displays and banged her head on the mother's leg. The parent often asked Natalie to stop the misbehavior, but did not follow through on her warnings. Therefore, it appeared that the youngster's most problematic behavior, and the one that occurred most frequently, was aggression.

The *parenting style* appeared to be permissive-indulgent, with the mother being very nurturing and communicative with the child. In fact, she was too wordy, and also took what Natalie said at face value, attributing adult-like intent to her verbalizations. Maturity demands and control were low, based on report and observation. The mother also indicated that she sometimes felt depressed. Natalie's biologic father sees the youngster periodically, but on an inconsistent basis. The child's temperament appeared to resemble a slow-to-warm-up profile.

Consider Other Issues Other issues include the mother being overwhelmed by the demands of her job and single parenting, inconsistency between households, and, in particular, the need for attention on the part of the child (and competition with siblings). It also appears that the preschool reinforces Natalie's behavior by calling her mother and sending the child home (which she finds reinforcing).

Define Positive Behavior The desired positive behavior to be focused upon is not hitting, kicking, throwing objects, screaming, pinching, or being destructive to objects in the home. This was termed a "temper tantrum" by the mother and explained to the child.

Plan for Problem Behavior A four-minute time-out was to be employed whenever the defined temper tantrum occurred. If there was just yelling or stomping, one warning was to be delivered. In the case of actual physical aggression, no warning would be provided, with the time-out being instituted immediately. If there was no time-out given for the problem behavior that day, then Natalie could put a sticker on a calendar and was then entitled to one-on-one "special time" with her mother. A reward menu was developed, containing special time activities such as reading a book, rough and tumble play, braiding her hair, or playing a simple board game. Watching television or a movie generally is not a good special time activity. If the child accumulated a total of four stickers (not necessarily in a row), then a larger, more long-term reward such as a trip for ice cream, fast food, or a special activity, could be employed.

Follow-up This program could then be expanded to involve the volitional daytime wetting. This was addressed by use of a grab-bag for not wetting, and overcorrection (i.e., cleaning up) when the child voided in her pants. The initial short-term reinforcement for reduction in tantrums was selected because it also addressed the attention-seeking motivation to the child's misbehavior, and also enhanced the parent-child interaction. The grab bag was employed in the scaffolding behavioral program to keep it distinct from the temper tantrum intervention. In fact, interventions geared to decrease temper displays will often also extend to other problem behaviors as well, and one would expect that the wetting would also decrease to some extent without being addressed specifically.

Several environmental or situational risks exist, these being a single mother, limited social support, fatigue, and possible depression. Protective factors include nurturance, communication, and motivation to change. Child risks include a slow-to-warm-up temperament. Natalie's brightness, cuteness, and desire for adult attention are protective factors. On the continuum of problem behaviors, the current situation appears to be more than a normal developmental variation, approaching the problem level; the severity is moderate.

General Principles There are several general principles that also can be distilled from the case. These principles underscore broader issues that are applicable to intervention with behavioral problems and include:

- *Address one behavior at a time.* The selected behavior should be one that occurs frequently and causes significant distress. This enables the parent to have better focus and more control over the intervention; this procedure also increases the likelihood of consistency.

- *Define the antecedent → behavior → consequence (ABC) chain.* In so doing, patterns of interaction are clarified, and the schedule of reinforcement/consequences can be elucidated. This process affords the opportunity to interrupt the non-productive chain of events more effectively.
- *Expand the scope of the intervention to other behaviors.* Once the initial problem is addressed, other problem behaviors can be dealt with. This can be accomplished either by adding the behavior on to the protocol in use, or initiating a parallel protocol. Care must be taken, however, not to make the intervention protocols too complex or confusing for the child. Excessive complexity also increases the possibility of inconsistency in the parent(s).
- *Identification of other issues is very useful.* In this case, pinpointing the desire for attention allows identification of more potent reinforcers that have a more far-reaching impact. Moreover, dealing with underlying issues in this fashion also enhances other areas of family functioning, and would decrease the likelihood of similar, attention-seeking problems in the future. While this would not be a strict behaviorist approach per se, in working with children and their families, this expanded framework is more effective.
- *Establish "parental presence."* This is a major issue. Caretakers must establish their credibility, and affirm their intent to change the problem behavior. Transmitting this message is perhaps the most critical component in the management of behavioral problems. This issue has major ramifications with regard to the parent-child interaction in general, and establishment of parental presence will ameliorate many low intensity problems before they breach the threshold and evolve into more prominent issues. Doing so also enhances the child's sense of security.
- *Identify external reinforcers that may maintain the problem behavior.* In this case, the preschool unwittingly reinforced the problem behavior by calling the child's mother and sending the child home. Therefore, whenever Natalie wanted to leave preschool and have time with her mother, she simply had to demonstrate tantrums and aggression.

CASE 2. BEDTIME PROBLEM

Sam is a 5½ year-old who refuses to sleep in his own bed. Initially, when sent to bed he would have numerous "curtain calls," (drink of

*water, bathroom, tummy hurts) essentially prolonging the bedtime
ritual by at least an hour. More recently, he insists that one of his
parents must lay down with him, and remain in his room until he
falls asleep. Sam typically wakes up over the course of the night and
slips into his parents' bed. His parents will occasionally awaken and
try to get Sam to go back to his own bed, but they complain that they
are tired and don't have the energy to deal with this. If they do
attempt to get him back into his own bed, Sam protests loudly, to
the point that he awakens his younger sibling, and potentially may
irritate neighbors in the adjoining apartment. The parents say that
they are concerned that Sam reaches a stage of panic when made to
go back to his own bed.*

Identify/Define Problem This is a fairly straightforward problem
in daily routine. The sleep problem appears to have evolved over time,
starting as multiple attempts to stay up by needing a drink of water, having to go to the bathroom, wanting to blow his nose, and similar ploys.
This suggests that the behavior is learned, and probably does not reflect
"panic" per se. However, having the parents specifically delineate problem behaviors was informative, and in actuality there are two related
issues: (1) not going to sleep without a parent present, and (2) not staying
in his own bed.

It becomes obvious that attempts to control this behavior have been
highly inconsistent at best. No difficulties are found with peers or in
school, and there have been no major changes or stresses in the household.
Family interactions seem appropriate but are somewhat permissive, and
there does not appear to be a sibling issue causing the problem, as the
younger sibling goes to bed earlier in a separate room. The onset of the
bedtime issues does not correspond to birth of the sibling. Sam does not
have any identifiable risks.

While it typically is recommended that one behavior be addressed
at a time, because of the interrelatedness of the two issues, in this
case there are three options, namely, have the child go to sleep by himself,
have him stay in his bed throughout the night, or require Sam to go to
bed without a parent present *and* stay there. Because of the sequence of
events, (not going to sleep by himself is the first behavior in the chain of
events), the initial intervention should address this. However, this might
produce an increase in his refusal to stay in his own bed during the night.
After discussion with both parents, it was decided to address the
going to sleep issue first. If, however, there were an increase in Sam
coming into the parents' bed, then this would have to be addressed
simultaneously.

Consider Other Issues As a general rule, sibling issues must be considered, because in numerous situations, competitiveness, jealousy, or perceived displacement by a younger sibling can foster sleep problems in an older sibling. Sibling issues do not appear to be a major contributing factor in this case. Problems among the parents also must be considered in the treatment of sleep problems, as the need for one parent to stay with the child until he or she falls asleep disrupts the parents' own bedtime routine, as does introduction of the child during the night. In such instances, the parent role supercedes the spouse role; whether this is an intentional "excuse" to avoid intimacy, or the result of the child running the household, needs to be explored. If there are parental intimacy problems, then the likelihood of successfully eliminating the sleep disorder is decreased markedly. (Marital problems were not an issue in this case.) One must also determine the typical bedtime schedule. As a rule, highly variable schedules have a greater propensity for producing sleep problems. This was the case with Sam.

Define Positive Behavior The goal selected for the initial program is to have Sam go to bed on his own. The parents first need to transmit the message that it is *expected* that Sam will go to bed by himself. Employing maturity themes (big boys do this, this will allow you to go to sleepovers) also is helpful.

Program for Problem Behavior The parents need to be forewarned about the possibility of the extinction burst phenomenon, whereby Sam may initially increase the number of "curtain calls" or heighten their intensity when he is sent to bed. Because the parents sat with Sam approximately 30 to 45 minutes (sometimes as much as 60 minutes) before he went to sleep, rather than abruptly terminating the procedure and increasing the likelihood of a major protest, the parents would gradually decrease the duration of this activity.

Extinction Sam is told that from this point onward, the parents will stay with him only for 15 minutes and that he will go to sleep in his own bed. A timer will be set for this purpose. A set bedtime will also be established (this also includes weekends), with reasonable flexibility for special occasions. Weekends should also be included because two nights of disruption in the schedule will require several nights for readjustment in order to get Sam back into the routine. If Sam cries after the 15 minutes have elapsed, this behavior should not be reinforced. The child's requests, pleas, or whining should not be acknowledged. He could be given the option that if the crying doesn't stop, then the door will be closed. With younger children a subsequent 15-minute "check-in" could be implemented, with subsequent check-ins being 30 minutes later, 45 minutes, and so on. In Sam's case, this procedure was optional, but not strongly recommended, due to the fact that this might inadvertently reinforce the problem behavior.

The procedure should be implemented on a weekend, so that the family will not be disrupted on an evening preceding a work-day, and also to minimize inconvenience to the neighbors. In this situation, it would be helpful to inform the neighbors what is going on and perhaps offer them a bottle of wine in gratitude for their patience. If a sibling shares the same room, moving the child temporarily to the parents' bedroom (in a sleeping bag) may be necessary. This option has the added benefit of using normal sibling competition—if Sam's crying promotes *his sibling* sleeping in the bedroom with the parents, but not him, there is a decreased likelihood that Sam will continue this behavior solely for the sibling's benefit.

Rewarding Positive Behavior Conversely, positive behavior, namely going to sleep on his own, will need to be reinforced. Given that parental attention appears to be a potent issue in the genesis and maintenance of the problem behavior, this can also be used to enhance the likelihood of positive behavior. There are several components to the reward program:

- Every night that Sam goes to bed without protest earns him 20-minutes of *special time* with one of his parents the next evening, prior to going to bed. Various activities can be listed in an a priori fashion, such as reading, playing a board game, rough and tumble activity, working on a model or puzzle, and so on. This will be the short-term reward.
- A coupon will be given the morning after a successful bedtime routine has occurred. This can be redeemed for a long-term reward. Options (e.g., having a friend sleep over, renting a video, going for ice cream) should be listed on a reward menu.
- Once the program is set and is working, the time the parents spend in the bedtime ritual is decreased by 2 minutes every several nights, until it is eliminated (fading procedure).
- Contingency plans should also be outlined. If the use of positive reinforcement and shaping is not successful, and it is ascertained that the program is being followed, then a consequence or penalty can be connected with the continued crying (in addition to the extinction and reward for positive behavior). Loss of television or computer time the next day is a possible option.

Follow-up It is not unusual for the child to spontaneously begin to remain in bed through the night after the initial bedtime routine has been established. If this is not the case, then chaining *staying in bed* with *going to sleep without protest* (and a parent being present) can be implemented. Basically, this involves the parents now employing the same reinforcement procedure (and, possibly, penalties) when Sam demonstrates both desired behaviors. A shaping procedure can be employed here as well: if Sam does come into the parents' bedroom during the night, he is required to sleep in a sleeping bag that is situated at the foot of the bed. This will gradually be moved closer toward the door, into the hallway, and so on. Oftentimes, children will simply remain in their own bed, once they realize that they will not be able to sleep in the parents' bed any further. This intervention requires that the parents *consistently* not allow Sam to get into bed with them and may include use of some method to wake them up if the child comes into their room (including possibly closing their door).

As mentioned previously, in this case, no child or environmental risks can be identified. The parents are motivated to change and this is a positive factor. On the behavioral concern continuum, the child's behavior is a problem and not a disorder, and is of a moderate severity.

General Principles Once again, there are several general principles that can be extracted from this case and applied to sleep problems as well as other, more general behavioral concerns. These include:

- *Children should go to sleep in their own bed.* A red flag for bedtime problems is the situation in which the child goes to sleep in the parents' arms (in the case of younger children), on the couch, or in a sibling's bed and then is subsequently placed in their own bed after falling asleep. If this is the case, when the child awakens, she often is disoriented or fearful because this is not the place where she had fallen to sleep. Falling asleep with the television on also is problematic, as oftentimes the child becomes interested in the show that is on and is even more resistant to going to sleep. This also sets up a potential, non-productive bedtime ritual that can be long-term.
- *Siblings can be used to help modify a child's problem behavior.* Normal sibling rivalry, modeling, or having the sibling receive reinforcement and the child not receiving such can be potent additions to a basic behavior management program. In this case, the misbehavior actually facilitates the sibling sleeping in the parents' room.
- *Emphasizing that it is the parents' expectation that the child will overcome the targeted behavior problem is important.* This should be coupled with implicit maturity demands to help alter the child's mindset regarding the behavior that is being addressed.
- *Parents should anticipate an "up-front load" with regard to the problem behavior when an intervention is implemented.* Protest and intensification of the problem behavior actually are indicative of the fact that the intervention is working. Similarly, it generally

takes an *average* of two weeks to change an established bedtime problem; some children will require more time, while others will necessitate a shorter intervention.

- *Practitioners should evaluate the situation for a potential stressor whose presence is contiguous with the onset of the problem* (this was not the case with Sam). While a behavioral program similar to that outlined above would still be advisable if a stressor is identified, it also would be necessary to address the stressor as well.

- *Environmental engineering should be employed in the development of contingency plans* (e.g., in this case, picking a weekend, moving the sibling, perhaps alerting neighbors). Similarly, minimizing outside noise (but not having other family members go to extremes to maintain quiet) is advised. Other "perks" that alter the sequence of events or environmental cues should be considered, such as introduction of a night light, lava lamp, fiber optic lamp, or relaxing CD music (ambient or classical—not rap).

- *In certain situations, two behaviors may be highly interrelated and both might need to be addressed simultaneously* (e.g., going to sleep and staying in bed; temper tantrums and aggression). In such situations, it is not a contradiction to the general principle of picking one target behavior, as long as both interrelated issues occur together and can be tied to the same intervention program. Although it generally is easier to focus on one specific behavior, in some cases, reduction of one behavior might produce intensification of a corresponding behavior. Here it is appropriate to address both. Care must be taken to not make the program too complex or to include unrelated behaviors at the outset of an intervention program (this increases the likelihood of inconsistency).

- *Sleeping problems often are early indicators of later relationship disturbances.* These behaviors may be early indicators of a tendency toward anxiety and/or depression. Practitioners must also appreciate parental fears and concerns such as perceiving the child to be "vulnerable," and their readiness to take control of their child's behavior.

CASE 3. TIME-OUT REFUSAL

Louie is a 4-year-old child who tends to be aggressive. When reprimanded and sent to time-out, he refuses to stay seated, and essentially loses control. Louie demonstrates similar problems in his early childhood classroom. Louie has a language disorder and it is

extremely difficult to understand him. His parents are questioning
what would be the best type of disciplinary technique.

Identify/Define Problem The basic problem faced by the parents is
that Louie does not accept a time-out and remain there. The youngster
does not sit, runs away from time-out, and when told to return or is
escorted back to time-out, he screams, flails, and the parents often have to
restrain him. After he does so, the parents often become exasperated and
let things slide. They also have a difficult time determining whether Louie
truly understands the time-out procedure.

Consider Other Issues This situation is complicated by the child's
language disorder. While Louie has a documented articulation and verbal
expressive problem, there is the strong possibility of a receptive disorder
as well. This possibility is supported by parental report as well as the
clinician's observation that Louie does not seem to understand questions
posed to him, often giving rather tangential answers. This case underscores the quandry indicated earlier in this chapter, namely whether this is
volitional or due to a developmental problem. The parents infer this in
their mention of their confusion regarding how much Louie comprehends
about the disciplinary procedure. However, here the parents do not truly
appreciate the overlap between the behavioral problem and the identified
communication disorder. In fact, many children with communication disorders are aggressive because they are frustrated by their inability to carry
on a dialogue or get their point across; as a result, they resort to physical
means. Moreover, on the receptive end, if the child does not understand
the association between a misbehavior and a consequence, the confusion
could lead to out-of-control behavior.

Define Positive Behavior At this point, the desired behavior is for
Louie to comply with the time-out procedure. Even though in the causal
sequence, it is the aggressive behavior that is truly problematic and it is
the first step in the evolution of the undesired behavior, by not accepting a time-out, there is no deterrent to the initial aggressive behavior.
Therefore, although not readily apparent, if the child associates aggression
with acquisition of a time-out, and the time-out is effective as a negative
consequence to the aggression, then the time-out procedure should lead to
a decrease in aggression.

Describe Program Particular care must be taken to explain the
program in simple, but specific terms, more so in Louie's case because of
the communication problem. Aggression needs to be defined for Louie
so that he understands why he is being disciplined or given a time-out.
This should help to decrease the confusion Louie experiences and which
may cause him to become even more frustrated. He is to be given

a 4 to 5-minute time-out whenever a previously defined aggressive action occurs. The first choice will be to remain in the time-out chair. If Louie refuses and flees, then a step-up procedure will be employed, whereby he will be escorted ("manually guided") to his room. The door will be left open, but if Louie escapes, then the next step-up would be for the parent to hold the door closed. Environmental engineering should be employed, namely, all toys are to be removed from the room, as should breakable objects. A timer should be employed and at the end of the time-out, a one-sentence explanation of the reason for time-out should be offered to Louie. By no means should Louie be rewarded for staying in time-out, nor should he be held by a parent in the time-out chair.

Follow-up Once Louie complies with the time-out procedure, the main focus of the intervention can shift to the actual precipitating aggression. In addition to negative consequences, the grab-bag model of reinforcing appropriate behavior (no aggression which then means no time-outs) can then be implemented in conjunction with a long-term reward program. If Louie goes the entire day without a time-out he receives a grab-bag with an additional long-term reward as well. Also, Louie's language problem needs to be addressed in his early childhood education program, and it would be advisable for his parents to also enroll him in an extracurricular speech/language therapy program at the local hospital.

In this case, there is a definite child risk factor, namely, a communication disorder. Undoubtedly, this has a direct bearing on the behavioral problem. No environmental risks could be identified. His parents are nurturing, high in communication, but a bit weak in control and maturity demands (the latter undoubtedly influenced by the child's communication problem). The behavioral concern is more than a normal developmental variation, and appears to be a mild to moderate problem, due in part to the fact that it is happening at school as well.

General Principles Once again there are several general points that can be gleaned from this case.

- *Certain behavioral problems tend to have a higher probability in the presence of specific identified disorders*. This has been termed a "behavioral phenotype" (Aylward, 1997). Therefore, the practitioner needs to be cognizant of what types of behavioral problems are associated with defined disorders such as ADHD (e.g., impulsivity, immediate need for gratification), communication disorders (aggression, impulsivity), non-verbal learning disabilities (poor social awareness), or others.
- *When the child demonstrates risk factors* (in Louie's case, a communication disorder), *the behavioral intervention should take this*

into consideration and efforts to establish competencies in the area of risk (e.g., better communication skills) *should go hand in hand with the behavioral program.* With better communication skills, the child is less likely to resort to physical, aggressive behavior to resolve conflicts. This is often the case with learning disabilities. In certain situations, such as with ADHD, medication can help control symptoms and enhance the child's ability to benefit from efforts to develop competencies.

- *When addressing the chain of events in the problem behavior, a thorough analysis of the problem is necessary, and going back to the initial link in the chain is not always the best course of action* (in this case, addressing the time-out compliance before focusing on the aggression per se).

CASE 4. TOILETING PROBLEM

Laura is a 5-year-old who refuses to have a bowel movement on the toilet. Instead, she insists that her mother provide her with a diaper when she feels the need to defecate. Her mother typically then disposes of the diaper and cleans Laura. If the child is not provided with a diaper she launches into a temper tantrum, and refuses to have a bowel movement. She also has begun to demonstrate a "fear" of sitting on the toilet for a bowel movement, although she has no problem urinating on the toilet. Laura is in kindergarten, and hasn't had a problem with toileting there, this attributable to the fact that she refuses to go to the bathroom in school. Laura is argumentative with her parents, and occasionally, with her teacher as well. She is reported to be bossy with peers.

Identify/Define Problem In attempting to specify the problem behavior, it becomes apparent that the toileting issue may be but one manifestation of a proneness toward oppositional behavior. Laura was noted to be very demanding in the waiting room and essentially refused to come into the examination room, despite numerous maternal requests to do so. In fact, the mother was observed to ask Laura if she wanted to come into the room, basically setting the stage for a negative response. Both the mother and father are highly nurturing, and admitted to following through with consequences for misbehavior approximately 50% of the time. They also tended to explain at great length why the behavior was not desirable. Rather than have a conflict with their daughter, the parents often simply overlook mild to moderate intensity problematic behavior. Analysis of the behavioral pattern also suggested that Laura was quite demanding, oppositional, and controlling; on the positive side (protective) she is cute, bright, highly verbal, and has parents who are involved. It also was noteworthy, that although the child seemed to fear the toilet when placed there in order to have a bowel movement, she had no problem voiding. This underscores the learned nature of the behavior, and the associative chaining that has taken place (i.e., the toilet has now been associated with the bowel movement struggle).

The selected target behavior was to eliminate the child having a bowel movement in a diaper.

Consider Other Issues One consideration is a permissive parenting style. Second, there is the need to define when the toileting issue evolved and if there were any traumatic incidents that may have prompted the onset of the problem. It was determined that the toileting issue had been in existence for quite some time, even after the child developed bowel control. Moreover, there is no younger sibling whose introduction into the household might have prompted regressive behavior in Laura. Obviously, there has been no concerted attempt at changing the behavior, as the parents reported that the child's pediatrician told them to simply not make it an issue, and the problem will spontaneously resolve. Unfortunately, that was almost two years ago.

Define Positive Behavior The end result or goal of the intervention is for Laura to have a bowel movement on the toilet and not in her diaper. Obviously, this cannot be accomplished in one fell swoop, as the behavior has existed for quite some time. Therefore, a shaping procedure is required.

Describe Program The first step in the shaping protocol is to have Laura sit on the toilet several times each day without a diaper. This is in the hope of having her spontaneously have a bowel movement while sitting. She is not frightened of sitting on the toilet per se, as is evident in the fact that she has no problem voiding. Subsequently, she would need to sit on the toilet after she has requested a diaper in anticipation of a bowel movement. At first, the lid is closed and the young lady can be fully clothed. The next step would be to have the toilet lid open with Laura sitting on the seat in the diaper. She can read, listen to a boom-box, or color while seated. She then will need to sit on the toilet in the diaper with her pants down. With each step, if the young lady is compliant, she receives a sticker that is then placed on the calendar. Three stickers can be redeemed for a trip to the grab-bag; if Laura makes a good effort that day, she is also entitled to 20 minutes of special time with either of her parents (this is considered a demonstration of appreciation and positive regard from the parents). After she has a bowel movement in her diaper, she is required to remove it, place it in a sealed receptacle, and clean herself off with a shower massage, after her parent has turned the water on and adjusted the temperature. There is no "punishment" per se.

The next step in the program involves Laura having the diaper put on loosely by the parent prior to her sitting on the toilet; then the diaper is left unfastened (with the adhesive strip removed). If necessary, the diaper subsequently can then actually be placed in the toilet, so that Laura has a bowel movement *on* the diaper versus *in* it. Each successive approximation is rewarded with a sticker. The message of being a "big girl" is transmitted frequently. Once the program has been successful, and the success has been sustained, then the parents can simply "run out" of diapers and refuse to go get more.

There is a parallel program that should be in effect also, namely, the parents being less permissive and compliant in response to Laura's other demands. The issue here is that the parents need to establish "parental presence" and demonstrate in a calm, reassuring manner that they are in control. Once again, this provides structure and predictability, and affords reassurance to the child. Along these lines, if the child displays temper tantrums, these should be dealt with by use of time-outs (after one warning). Once parents establish credibility on this front, it has a greater likelihood of influencing Laura's response to the toileting intervention. This approach will also directly address the oppositional tendencies in the child, and the proclivity toward permissiveness in the parents.

Follow-up Obviously, if withdrawal of the diapers is met with refusal to toilet, then a high fiber diet, mineral oil, or a similar stool softener could be used under the direction of the child's primary care physician. Similarly, if Laura then resorted to having bowel movements in her pants or on the carpet, then consequences (cleaning the carpet or underwear in an overcorrection procedure) in conjunction with response cost (e.g., loss of movies, television viewing time) would be warranted.

In this case, permissive parenting is an environmental or situational risk factor. Child risks include oppositional tendencies and the fact that this behavior has existed for some time. Optimistic indicators include the fact that the child can urinate on the toilet, there are no problems when she is sleeping, and this has not become a problem at school. Therefore, the child has more control over this issue than initially was realized. On the continuum of behavioral concerns, it is a problem of moderate intensity, although there is the definite potential for this to evolve into encopresis, which indeed is a disorder.

General Principles There are several general points that can be extrapolated from this case:

- *With elimination problems (also in the development of toilet training), care must be taken to not place excessive, undue emphasis on the toileting issue.* Many families go overboard in their focus on the problem, and the added attention and control enjoyed by the child may evolve into a potent reinforcer. Therefore, the problem should be addressed in a matter-of-fact, but firm manner.
- *While addressing a specific problem, it is helpful to look at broader, related issues.* In this case, oppositional tendencies and permissive parenting interact and maintain the specific behavioral problem. Addressing these factors in the context of the behavioral intervention for the specific target behavior is recommended.
- *If the behavioral problem is of a passive-aggressive nature, punishment or shaming will only escalate the conflict, and therefore should be avoided.* Punishment, particularly if it is severe, will lead to resentment and, perhaps shame. Either of these sequelae might, consciously or unconsciously on the part of the child, maintain the behavior.
- *Once a problem behavior has been established, particularly avoidance behavior, shaping must be employed to alter it.* It is not realistic to expect a total, immediate change in a non-desirable behavior. Just as the problem behavior developed gradually and in incremental steps, its treatment should progress in the same manner. This must be explained to the parents at the outset of the intervention, so as to prevent unreasonable expectations.

CASE 5. HOMEWORK PROBLEM

Ralph is an 8-year-old third grader who has a large amount of homework each night. Over the last 6 months, homework sessions have evolved into a lengthy, nightly ordeal that distresses not only Ralph, but his entire family as well. The homework conflicts frequently extend late into the evening, and often result in screaming, crying, and resentment. This situation has had a negative impact on Ralph's grades and his teacher has suggested the possibility of retention.

Identify/Define Problem This type of problem occurs in many households. Basically, Ralph is reluctant to sit down and do his homework, and this has evolved into avoidance-type behavior. He simply does not perceive that it is far easier to complete the homework, both in terms of time and also problems the next day, than to attempt to avoid doing so. Although homework is an aversive stimulus, it is not clear as to why this is the case. The sequence of the problem behavior begins with the mere mention of homework, which essentially is the trigger for the ensuing course of events. This is a conditioned response, and while it is helpful to consider reasons why this has become conditioned, it is not essential to do so. Once the sequence begins, Ralph's ability to focus on homework is precluded by the highly emotionally charged situation. Moreover, the behavior is reinforced on a partial reinforcement schedule, in that there are times that the conflict has extended late into the evening, without the homework being completed.

Consider Other Issues While consideration of other issues may deviate from the strict behavioral approach, a more complete understanding of this type of problem is extremely helpful in dealing with the undesirable behavior. There are several issues that often contribute to the child not doing homework. Questions exploring these issues include:

- *Is the amount of homework reasonable?* Excessive amounts of homework could be the result of a hard-driving teacher, an educational institution that prides itself in high academic achievement, or work that was not completed in class. Parents are advised to check with parents of classmates to ascertain which of the options is most likely.
- *Does the child have an attention deficit hyperactivity disorder, particularly the inattentive subtype?* This could make it difficult for the child to complete work in the classroom and then have an additional, negative impact on his ability to sit down to do homework later in the day.
- *Does the child have a learning disability?* If this is the case, then the child has had to work doubly hard during the day to deal with material that is made more difficult by the learning problem, and again has to address the same problem later on in the evening. This is particularly the case with a significant reading disability. To some children, refusing to do homework, that is, asserting that "I won't do it" is more face-saving than admitting, "I can't do it."
- *Does the homework scenario afford the child individual attention from the parents or allow her to take control of the family evening activities?* Alternatively, if a child takes on the "problem role," this may divert family conflict onto the child, versus having the intactness of the family threatened.

- *Is the child having social difficulties in school?* If peers are picking on him routinely, the child may simply not be able to focus on classroom work and therefore has to bring it home. Similarly, the homework will then be associated with school, and school is the last thing the child wants to deal with once he returns home.
- *Is the task presented in a manner that is overwhelming for the child?* Placing a pile of papers in front of the child, and requiring him to sit at a table until it is completed is less effective than breaking the homework time into study blocks of 20-minutes each, with specified amounts of work to be done during that interval.

Define Positive Behavior The target behavior is to have Ralph complete his homework in a timely, non-confrontational manner.

Describe the Program A shaping procedure is necessary, in which the parents and teacher need to work together to initially reduce the amount of work, so as to allow the child to experience success. A set amount of work will need to be completed in a specific time frame. There will be allotted breaks during the homework time period. Obviously, the amount of work and duration of the homework session will be determined by delineating some of the causative factors listed above.

Moreover, if Ralph complies with the stipulations that have been selected, he should be given a reinforcement. A helpful technique is the coupon approach in which at the successful completion of a round of homework, Ralph is given a coupon. Coupons can be redeemed for a variety of rewards of different values that are listed on a reward menu. For example, 5 coupons could be redeemed for a video rental, 10 coupons for a sleepover, and so on. Bonus coupons could be doled out if Ralph has 5 successful rounds in a row or if a homework session went particularly well. This can be expanded to include a larger reward, whereby Ralph would be eligible for a second tier reinforcement once he had achieved a cumulative, running total of perhaps 30 coupons (even though he might have cashed them in previously for smaller rewards). Alternating which parent helps him, as well as considering having a tutor at least one night per week, are two additional components that have been found to be useful. This same approach can be employed if a child needs to work on areas of academic difficulty (e.g., use of a computer program to enhance reading) in addition to regular schoolwork, or is academically weak and needs to remain current in certain subjects over the summer months. With older children, a point system could be employed instead of the use of coupons, but the same basic reinforcement approach would apply.

Follow-up Once the homework pattern is established, the amount can be increased somewhat, but care must be exercised to not overload the youngster. Without doubt, the etiology of the avoidance behavior needs to be addressed as well. If another child with similar problems is identified, and the parents are familiar to each other, buddy homework sessions could be explored. Here, one set of parents is responsible for both children completing their homework on odd-numbered days, and the other parents would have the homework sessions at their house on even-numbered days. This affords respite for each family, and also makes the homework session more enjoyable for the children, particularly if playtime is scheduled to occur at the end of the session.

In this case, the potential for a child risk factor (e.g., ADHD, learning disability) is increased. Because we are dealing with avoidance behavior, there most likely is a causal chain, and this needs to be identified. There do not appear to be situational risks, although it is not certain as to the reasons for the large amount of homework. The behavioral concern is moderate to severe, but would only escalate if not addressed in a timely fashion. More specifically, because the child would not work on academics, he would fall further behind. This would produce an increased amount of homework, which, in turn, would cause further avoidance. This vicious cycle would intensify. Punishment should not be the initial intervention technique, but response cost could also be employed (e.g., loss of television that night) as an adjunct to the coupons, if the homework refusal is more volitional (and not due to significant learning or attention problems) and the child is not responding to a more positive approach.

General Principles Once again, there are several general principles that can be extracted from the case.

- *When a school situation has an impact on home, etiologies at both ends need to be investigated.* This is particularly the case with homework. The U.S. Department of Education (1992) reported, "parents are the earliest, and can be the most consistent and proximal, influence in establishing and supporting lifelong learning" (p. B-20). It has been recommended that elementary school students be assigned one hour of homework per night (less at lower elementary grades; e.g., 20 minutes per night in first grade, increasing by 10 minutes per grade), and at least 2 hours for high school students, although these guidelines are open to significant debate. Homework does appear to be moderately advantageous in terms of school achievement, but there are special considerations if a child has a learning or attention disorder. In general, parents should have a *supportive* role with regard to homework, versus function as instructors or tutors (Roderique, Polloway, Cumblad, Epstein, & Bursuck, 1994). The supportive role includes providing sufficient space and time for homework completion, monitoring task completion, and allocating a specific time period for homework. Maintenance-type (versus acquisition-type) homework tasks that involve practice and completion are generally less problematic (particularly for children with learning or attention problems), while class preparation and extension activities could produce more conflict.

- *By no means should a child have so much homework that there is absolutely no time for other pursuits.* There are numerous situations in which a child does homework after school until suppertime, and then from after supper until bedtime during the week. Add to this Sunday afternoon and evening. This schedule precludes participation in any extracurricular activities or even the ability to simply play, and increases the likelihood of emotional sequelae. Such scenarios are frequently encountered in children with unidentified learning or attention problems, where teachers or school administrators do not allow for modifications or accommodations, instead implying that the child is "lazy."

- *Excessive parental involvement in homework is a red flag for an underlying problem.* If the child can obtain decent grades, but must participate in the vicious "dawn-to-dusk" academic cycle outlined above in order to obtain these grades, then further evaluation of underlying issues is necessary. This academic treadmill will continue to go faster and faster until the child (and parents) simply cannot keep up once the academic demands increase (usually from 3rd to 5th grade).

- *Retention is not an effective intervention.* Retention without specific interventions geared toward addressing the causes for academic difficulty borders on negligence. Unfortunately, retention in early grades is common and, in fact is increasing in many communities (Byrd & Weitzman, 1994). It is estimated that nationally, 7.6% of children have repeated kindergarten or first grade. Early grade retention has not been proven effective in improving learning and it has a significant, negative impact on a child's self-esteem, and attitude toward school. Many children view retention as punishment or a sign of failure (Shepard & Smith, 1989). Grade retention also increases the risk of subsequent school drop-out (Byrd & Weitzman, 1994). Retention implies "catch-up," but catch-up is not supported in the literature. Any initial gains from the retention year wash out quickly, and children who are deemed "immature" (a frequently cited "cause" for repeating a grade) do not benefit from and extra year to "grow." In fact, children who are younger at school entry are not at increased risk for retention in early grades when compared to peers who were older at school entry. Academic "red-shirting" therefore is not productive. The practice of retention is analogous to running a race with a broken leg and coming in last. Instead of fixing the leg, the child is told to run the same race once again, most likely again coming in last. Stated differently, a problem in learning is still a problem, regardless of grade retention. Moreover, children with certain characteristics have a greater likelihood of grade retention. These characteristics include low socio-economic status, male gender, low maternal education, hearing or speech deficits, behavioral problems, having been born low birth weight (<2500 g), or having been exposed to household smoking. Conversely, high maternal education and residing with both biological parents at age 6-years are associated with a decreased risk of retention (Byrd & Weitzman, 1994). Retention in later grades is a particularly misguided undertaking, and if a youngster is retained in middle school or later, the likelihood of emotional sequelae and a complete academic shutdown is increased dramatically. If retention is *absolutely* necessary, such as in the case of a child moving from a school system with low academic standards to one with exceptionally high levels, then this must be done in earlier grades; physical size (especially in males), age close to cut-off, academic delays not being severe, and lack of opportunity for adequate instruction are concerns that *may*, in isolated cases, support retention.

CASE 6. PROBLEM WITH SEPARATION

Katie is a 3-year-old who displays an intense reaction whenever she separates from her mother. She refuses to stay with a sitter, even if the sitter is one of her grandparents. More recently, she even refuses to go to her father when he calls her, or stay with him while her mother runs errands. When held by her father, Katie cries and protests that she wants her mommy, this often occurring in front of family friends and relatives. Katie's mother has stated that her daughter has always been "determined" and is verbally precocious.

Identify/Define Problem This behavioral concern is of an avoidant/overdependent type, and most likely has been reinforced. It appears that Katie's mother has been compliant with regard to her daughter's demands, and therefore the behavior has worsened. A particularly pertinent question involves whether the mother sees this behavior as a problem, or, instead interprets it as being indicative of close attachment. If it is the latter, the likelihood of successfully implementing the intervention is reduced. Similarly, it is important to gauge how the grandparents and the father respond to the child's behaviors. In this type of situation, it is best to interview both parents together and have them independently develop a list of the 3 most problematic behaviors. In this case, it would appear that separation from the mother is the common denominator.

Consider Other Issues This type of behavior sometimes occurs in the presence of parental conflict, vis á vis "detouring" (where the conflict between the parents is detoured through the child, rather than have them be directly confrontational). It would be helpful to informally assess the possibility of a mother-daughter coalition that essentially excludes the father. Moreover, if this is the case, it is important to evaluate generational boundaries that separate the mother and daughter roles, taking care to determine whether the boundaries are blurred. The possibility of a vulnerable child status is also raised, and it also is useful to ascertain whether there is a positive family history for depression or anxiety (although Katie's age would make a genetic basis rather unlikely at this time). In the past, such behavior was considered *symbiotic*, but viewed pragmatically, symbiosis is bi-directional, with needs typically being met for both parties. It also appears that the behavior is unwittingly reinforced by giving in to the child, giving her attention, and perhaps even covert approval.

Define Positive Behavior The desired behavior is to have Katie not become upset upon separation from her mother, and to not protest when in the care of her father or other family members.

Describe the Program Given this type of behavioral problem, extinction would be the best approach. More specifically, all family members need to be in agreement that this behavior is not desired and could become more problematic in the future (i.e., when Katie enters preschool). Therefore, such behavior should not be considered "cute" nor should it be reinforced by allowing the child to have her way. Firm limits need to be set whereby if, for example, Katie cries in protest when picked up by her father, the mother should simply reaffirm that the child must indeed stay with dad, and not give any hint that she, herself, is distressed by the child's behavior. She (the mother), should then remove herself from the conflict. Attention to the behavior must be downplayed. Distraction might be used in the course of the extinction procedure, as could shaping. Use of positive reinforcement aside from praise or positive statements for the appropriate behavior is not recommended. Environmental engineering in which the mother runs an errand, leaving the child with her father or grandparents should be orchestrated. During these times, fun activities should be planned for the youngster.

Follow-up If it becomes apparent that Katie has a vulnerable child status, parent education as well as shaping of parental behavior will be necessary. If there are problems with the spousal subsystem, to the point that one or both spouses define their relationship solely in terms of the parent role, then concomitant couples counseling will be required. The practitioner might make the suggestion that the parents need to go out to dinner and have a sitter (initially a family member) watch Katie, with the additional stipulation that over the course of the evening their discussions should not involve their daughter. The goal here is to strengthen the spousal component of the executive subsystem. Similarly, the parents will need to support each other when dealing with any of Katie's problematic behaviors. Frequently in this type of situation, working on parallel issues (relationships) will improve the problem behavior (separation issues).

Modeling can also be employed if the mother has a friend with a child who is close in age to Katie. The mother can first leave Katie with her peer and the peer's mother in the family's home. This could then be expanded to have Katie stay at the friend's house.

While the magnitude of the problem behavior is mild to moderate, this type of concern can rapidly develop into a more serious issue, the longer it is reinforced. Moreover, there are strengths or protective factors in the child (e.g., precocious language abilities) but there are potential environmental risks in terms of parental interactions and permissiveness as well.

General Principles Once again there are several generalizations that can be extracted from this case:

- *In the presence of behavioral problems that seem to be divisive for the parents, potential causes for the conflict should be addressed in conjunction with behavioral interventions directed toward the child.* All too often, behavioral problems that cause friction among spouses are the offshoot of underlying, broader issues. Similarly, if the parental mindset is that the child is somehow medically vulnerable, the parents may direct all their energies into protecting the child, and acquiescing to her demands, this at the cost of maintaining their own relationship. While parents may initially resent probing into issues other than the child's identified problem, couching this inquiry in terms of more effectively doing what is best for the child often is more acceptable. Furthermore, if the underlying issues are not addressed, the likelihood of the behavioral problem being successful decreases substantially.
- *If a behavioral problem seems to disproportionately affect one of the parents, it is critical to evaluate how each perceives the*

problem and how each parent addresses it. Only in this manner can a better understanding of the magnitude and evolution of the problem behavior be obtained. This understanding will be critical in the formulation of an effective intervention strategy. Along these lines, appreciation of family dynamics such as detouring, triangulation, coalitions, boundaries, and spousal/parent roles, and ways to effectively alter these non-productive interchanges is necessary.

- *A child's behavioral predisposition can often serve as the vehicle for family conflict.* In Katie's case, her tendency toward being "determined", coupled with good verbal skills and perhaps some anxiousness, provide the basis for a detouring phenomenon. Had she been sickly early on or if she had a perceived life-threatening condition, then care of this problem might have been the major focus of the parents, with a resultant vulnerable child status evolving. Similarly, had Katie demonstrated externalizing, aggressive behavior, this behavior would then be the primary issue to preoccupy family interactions.
- *Parental reinforcement of a problem behavior can be conscious, unconscious, or simply done unwittingly.* Determination of which of these options is correct is difficult, but nonetheless extremely important, as the cause for the reinforcement, if not addressed, can render a strict behavioral approach ineffective.

CASE 7. REFUSAL TO DO CHORES

Keith is a 10-year-old youngster who has a significant articulation disorder. His parents, particularly the mother, complain that Keith is lazy and that he refuses to do any chores without protest or having the parents resort to yelling and threatening him with a loss of privileges. He would sit in front of the television the entire day if allowed to, and he spends a great deal of time on the internet and playing videogames. Keith's family did not bring him in earlier because his father had recently lost his job due to corporate downsizing. This also precluded the family from obtaining outside help with his articulation problem.

Identify/Define problem Keith has gotten to the point that he even has become lax with respect to personal hygiene and has to be constantly reminded to bathe, brush his teeth, or comb his hair. He does not throw out the trash, clean up after himself in the kitchen, pick up his room, mow the lawn, or bring his dirty laundry to the laundry room without protest.

Therefore, the basic problem is non-compliance with parental requests (demands), and acceptance of responsibility. The parents frequently state that they are going to take away privileges, but only do so when they are pushed to the limit. If Keith is told to have tasks completed by the time the parents get home from work, he usually prefers to watch television instead. After the parents arrive home and repeat their demands multiple times, he often eventually will comply, but under protest. He is more likely to comply if the father makes demands, but the father does so only sporadically. The mother is the main authority figure on a day-to-day basis. In this case, use of the list of the 3 most problematic, specific behaviors is essential, as "not listening" or "being lazy" are very difficult to operationalize.

Consider Other Issues There does seem to be a discrepancy regarding Keith's compliance to the mother and father's requests. He is more likely to take the father seriously. This could be due to the fact that the father is more consistent in doling out consequences, or simply because the father is less inconsistent due to the fact that he does not interact with Keith as much as his wife does. The mother typically makes numerous lists of things for Keith to do, and apparently she does this for her husband as well. The husband loathes such lists. Keith's articulation problems may make him prone to getting picked on by peers or upperclassmen. The loss of his father's job increases the possibility of family stress, which may have an indirect impact on Keith's behaviors (even thought these problems have existed prior to this situation). The articulation disorder may have a negative impact on the youngster's social interactions and this needs to be investigated.

Define Positive Behavior The desired behavior involves Keith complying with the parents' directives on the first request. This should be done without protest, and done appropriately.

Describe the Program It becomes apparent that Keith is on a variable ratio reinforcement schedule, meaning that he frequently gets away with not doing chores. In fact, it is "economically" better for him to be lax, protest, and not complete the tasks until he is forced to because: (a) there is a good chance that he will not have to do the task subsequently, and (b) there is no additional consequence that results from Keith not doing the task initially or protesting, even though he may eventually have to do the chore that was requested. Moreover, he rarely receives a consequence that matters, that is to say the parents do not stick to the penalties that they impose. Therefore, there should be two major components to the program. The first component involves having a consequence for not doing the requested task (and having some type of positive consequence if he does). The second component involves an additional consequence if there is an argument, protest, or avoidance of the task, even if Keith eventually does the chore.

Given the child's age, coupled with the need to not necessarily provide rewards for doing chores that are required simply as being a member of the family, the following intervention protocol was selected. First, Keith is given a weekly allowance, so this would be increased somewhat, and made contingent upon completing specified chores (e.g., $10.00 per week). The chores were specific: cleaning the kitchen area each day, throwing out the trash, picking up his jacket, shoes, and bookbag, and mowing the lawn when requested to do so. Each time a chore is not completed, $.50 would be deducted from initial allowance amount. If Keith argued about the chore, an additional $.25 would be deducted. Bonuses ($.25) could be given out at the parents' discretion for a particularly prompt or efficient job. These monetary values could be adjusted by the parents if it becomes apparent that Keith still has ample money left at the end of the week, even though he did not complete a sizeable number of chores. Moreover, he should not be given any additional money by the parents that may replace money lost by the program (that could be used to go to the movies or out with friends), as this would decrease the impact of the loss of money for non-compliant behavior. The program must be delivered on a consistent basis, and should be agreed upon by both parents.

Follow-up It often is the case that parents allow a child a bit more leeway if he or she has a developmental problem. In Keith's case, the articulation problem is significant, and the parents may feel somewhat guilty about the fact that they are unable to pursue extracurricular speech therapy (the school provides the routine 30-minutes per week). This problem may also make Keith vulnerable to being picked on by peers, particularly given his age. This, coupled with the early adolescent developmental level (adolescence begins at age 10-years), and the rejection of parental values and need to establish one's own identity, might cause Keith to become more passively rebellious. Similarly, the possibility of depression should be investigated, as "being different" is a major issue in early adolescence (even though this may be denied by Keith). The impact of the father's employment status on the spousal relationship and parenting practices also needs to be considered as this is a situational risk factor. It would also be advantageous for the parents to attempt to secure more speech-language intervention to deal with the stuttering. This is an effort to address the child risk factor and enhance a basic competency.

The severity of the problem behavior is mild to moderate. Nonetheless, it is causing a fair degree of stress in the household. Risk factors in the child include the articulation deficit and possible peer problems. Environmental risks include permissive parenting, parental disagreements regarding "lists," and the father's employment status and resultant family stress. In this case, normal developmental issues (i.e., early adolescence) also have a probable impact.

General Principles Generalizations from this case follow.

- *In the course of noncompliant behavior that eventually becomes compliant, the ancillary behavior associated with the noncompliance (e.g., protest, passive-aggressiveness) should also be followed by a consequence, even if the request is finally met by the child.* In many situations, the child will eventually comply with parental requests, but in the course of doing so he has displayed flagrant disregard and disrespect for the parents' wishes, may have been argumentative, and, in a sense, in control. While he has to eventually give in and do the chore, he would have had to do that anyway. Therefore, the misbehavior potentially could be reinforced because it has obviously caused the parents distress, and this show of noncompliance really did not cost the child anything above what would have occurred even if he did comply on the first request. Therefore, even in the face of eventual compliance, the initial noncompliance needs to have a consequence.

- *In the course of conceptualizing a behavioral concern, the practitioner and parent must consider developmental issues and the impact of external forces.* With Keith, early adolescence has certain developmental issues that may exacerbate the situation. More specifically, the need for peer acceptance, individuality, and questioning of parental values are typical, and, unfortunately fit into the current problem. This will be the case until age 13 or 14 years, whereupon the young man will then move into the middle stage of adolescence, which has its own, unique developmental conflicts and issues. From 5th to 8th grades, being picked on by peers reaches its highest level. This is a way for other young adolescents to impress their friends by picking classmates or others in school who are particularly vulnerable. Physical differences (taller, shorter, heavier, thinner, glasses, braces) as well as behavioral problems (stuttering, articulation problems, impaired gait, nervous mannerisms, tics, etc.) make a child particularly vulnerable to criticism. The negative effects of such criticism are particularly pronounced because the young adolescent is driven by the need for peer acceptance, and is attempting to develop a sense of self. This frustration may then emerge as an attempt to take control over a situation, even though the situation is not related to the underlying issue. Moreover, emotional distress that might result from peer issues could further exacerbate the need to exert some control, albeit non-productive.

- *Family stress due to external forces can exacerbate an existing behavioral problem.* One might use the metaphor of the family being similar to a ship that barely manages to stay afloat and whose bilge pumps are working overtime to accomplish this. If additional high seas start to batter the ship further (i.e., environmental stresses having an impact on family function), the precarious ability of the bilge pumps to maintain buoyancy may simply be overwhelmed. In Keith's case, the behavioral problems had existed previously, and the family was having problems to begin with. The loss of the father's job further depletes the parents' ability to channel energy to address the behavioral concern, and in fact, may help to maintain the behavior.

CASE 8. SCHOOL DIFFICULTY

Chloe is a 10-year-old who is not completing her work in school. Her grades have progressively declined and currently she is receiving D's and F's. She does not seem to care about school, and frequently complains of stomachaches that are vague and not accompanied by other positive indicators of illness. She is reluctant to do homework, but does comply with her parents' requests to complete it; unfortunately she often does not turn it in even if the work is completed. The teacher complains that Chloe "spaces out" frequently.

Identify/Define Problem The parents are in a quandary and complain of declining grades, Chloe not doing her work in school, and not turning her homework in, even if it is completed. They also are concerned about her physical complaints, which are more pronounced on schooldays. In addition, the parents also indicate that the teacher has brought up the possibility of an attention deficit hyperactivity disorder, the teacher reporting that she can spot this type of problem easily, because her own child has ADHD, and she has had numerous children in her classroom in the past with the disorder. The parents wonder if Chloe is simply lazy, because of her reluctance to invest energy into academics.

Consider Other Issues In selecting the target behavior, each of the complaints in the parents' list of most problematic behaviors needs to be considered, and it would be very helpful to identify a common cause if possible. In this situation, historical information is of utmost value, as it will help to determine whether this problem is due to a learning disorder, ADHD, or peer issues. With respect to the possibility of a learning disorder several types of information would be helpful: (1) report cards, paying close attention to patterns of grades and whether there has indeed been a decline (and if there has, whether it occurred at any specific time); (2) standardized testing such as the California Achievement Tests or Iowa Tests of Basic Skills, paying attention to percentiles or stanines (3–7 being the average range with respect to the latter); (3) samples of schoolwork, to evaluate carelessness, inability to follow directions, handwriting, and variability in performance. In general, if the report cards are suggestive of a precipitous drop in grades within the last year or two, the cause is probably not a learning disability. Similarly, if standardized testing indicates average or above average performance, the likelihood of a learning disability is also decreased. Conversely, if these scores are low, this could indicate a learning problem, an attention problem, or disinterest in the testing procedure. As it stands, Chloe's scores on standardized testing administered in the first, third and fifth grades were average; her report cards consisted of A's and an occasional B through third grade, with highly variable performance occurring thereafter.

With respect to ADHD, Chloe's teacher rating scale was positive (as would be expected, given the teacher's earlier statements), while the parent report, and a form from Chloe's Sunday School teacher were negative for ADHD symptoms. There was no mention of this concern in earlier grades, and there is no positive family history for such. The acceptable scores on standardized testing did not support this possibility either.

Peer relations were a definite possibility as a causative factor because of several characteristics. Chloe is a tall, somewhat overweight young lady with glasses. She is rather clumsy, and her interests with respect to toys and television shows are more similar to those of a 7- or 8-year old, than a female entering early adolescence. Her parents report little contact with peers outside of school, with Chloe's main social contact being a 7-year-old neighbor. Chloe rides the bus to and from school, and tries to wait until the last minute before going to the bus stop. Her stomachaches typically appear around the time she is to leave for school. Chloe's only sibling is almost 20 years old and is out of the house. When asked if she has lots of friends, a few friends, or "not too many," Chloe selected the last option.

Define Positive Behavior The desired behavioral outcome is obtaining adequate grades, defined as nothing lower than a "C."

Describe the Program This type of school problem necessitates excellent communication between the parents and teacher. It also will necessitate a multi-pronged approach. The parents will need to first converse with the teacher to delineate three or four of the most problematic behaviors that occur in the classroom. These can then be printed on a half-page form, and written in a positive, versus negative manner. More specifically, items selected to be checked by the teacher in boxes on the form were: (1) Chloe turned in her homework (versus Chloe did not turn in her homework); (2) Chloe completed most of her assigned work in class; (3) Chloe participated in class discussion; and (4) Chloe made a good effort in class. Chloe is required to bring this note home each day, signed by the teacher. Initially, in a shaping procedure, three out of four items should be checked in order for Chloe to receive a coupon (which then could be redeemed for items on a reward menu). Bonus coupons could be given for good grades on tests. Subsequently, all four items would need to be endorsed, and item number 2 would be reworded to delete, "most of."

Adjunctive components to the program include getting Chloe involved in social activities both in and out of school (as well as church), identifying possible protagonists in the classroom who may be bullying or isolating the young lady, and getting her involved in counseling that would focus on social skill development and conflict resolution. Because of the nature of the problem, it would be counterproductive to punish the young lady for poor school performance at this point.

Follow-up In securing the teacher's cooperation, it should be emphasized that she was indeed perceptive and helpful, but that the inattentiveness she detected was due to issues other than ADHD. This cooperation is critical in implementation of the program. In this situation it would not be productive to focus solely on grades per se, even though this is the major concern. Rather, placing emphasis on the individual components that contribute to the grades enhances a more functional cognitive mindset for Chloe. More specifically, demonstration of desirable classroom behavior is associated with reinforcement; the end result of this more positive classroom behavior is improvement in grades. However, the major issue still involves stress emanating from non-optimal peer interactions, and this emotional issue has a significant impact on Chloe's attitude toward school. Unfortunately, this is more difficult to address and requires broader intervention.

The severity of this problem is high, with the young lady doing extremely poorly in school and essentially placing herself in academic jeopardy. Loneliness, low self-esteem, depressed mood and risk for development of maladaptive behaviors exist. A significant rejection rate by peers unfortunately is a good predictor of later psychopathology and emotional disorders. While there are no environmental or situational risks within the family (aside from what appears to be a paucity of maturity demands), there are definite situational stressors in terms of peer interactions.

Chloe displays some characteristics that place her at risk, these including immature behaviors, a tendency to internalize stress and display somatic complaints, and physical characteristics that increase the possibility of ridicule from peers (even though there is no true basis for such ridicule). The possibility of depression should be investigated, although this overall situation appears to resemble an adjustment disorder. While participation in counseling is warranted, the practitioner can help to shore up Chloe's self-esteem a bit by being empathic, indicating that "good kids" are the ones that get picked on, and to allow her grades to slide simply allows the antagonists to "win," because it is Chloe getting into academic difficulty, and not them. Refocusing her anger in a more appropriate way (i.e., obtaining better grades) actually allows her to "win." Breaking the approach down into small components such as the items contained in the teacher checklist also makes the intervention appear more manageable to the young lady, who probably is overwhelmed with the enormity of the situation, and a sense of futility.

General Principles Again, there are several general tenets and techniques that can be extracted from this case. These include:

- *In cases where emotional issues that cause the problem behaviors are due to environmental stresses or situations external to the family (e.g., peer problems), interventions need to be multifaceted.* Simply emphasizing good grades and solely directing the intervention to improving grades, without addressing the day-to-day frustration and anger that the child experiences most likely will not be successful. Chloe most likely does contribute in some way to the situation (even though it most likely is not her fault), and changing how she interacts would definitely be a positive step. Hence, a social skills development group would be excellent, as would some individual therapy to bolster her self-confidence and self-esteem. Similarly, in this type of situation, employment of other activities to improve *competencies* (e.g., extracurricular peer activities) is necessary.
- *Bullying takes many forms, ranging from active, physical means to more passive, non-physical types.* Grades 5 through 8 are probably the most difficult times in terms of bullying of any type. While males typically employ physical means such as pushing, hitting, verbal aggression and threats, females use more passive measures such as exclusion, rumors, or derogatory verbal comments. Unfortunately, the latter seems to have a more long-term negative impact on the child's self-esteem, and it often is not as easy for a teacher to observe in the classroom or playground (although it

might be more obvious in the latter, when the child tends to be isolated).

- *Children judge their self-worth in terms of opinions of others.* Loss
  of self-esteem leads to inappropriate efforts to gain peer acceptance and becomes cyclical over time. This fact underscores why it
  is imperative for the practitioner and parents to not dismiss the
  potential severity of the problem and to address it as early as possible.
- *A child's level of social success should be identified.* If the child
  has the capacity to maintain one or two good friendships, this suggests that she has social skills, is successful in that regard, and in
  some cases, this is sufficient. Social skills per se are positive social
  behaviors that contribute to the initiation and maintenance of
  positive social interaction in context with peers.
- *Social skill questions should be posed to the child by the practitioner, and these would drive the type of intervention emphasized
  in counseling. These questions include*: (1) Do you have a lot of
  friends, a few friends, or not too many friends? (2) Are they close
  friends or acquaintances (i.e., see them only at school, or have
  additional contact); (3) Do you go on sleepovers or birthday parties? (4) Do some kids pick on you or do they ignore you (or both)?
  (5) What do kids pick on you about? (6) Do you get in fights a lot
  (do you start them)? (7) Are you lonely at school or at home?
  (8) What kinds of things do you like about yourself?/What kinds
  of things do you not like? (9) Do other kids think you're bossy?
- *Practitioners should also pose social skills questions to the parents
  regarding their child's behaviors.* Again, this would enable a better
  assessment of the problem behavior. These include: (1) Is your
  child bossy or aggressive? (2) How does your child do with friends?
  (3) Does your child avoid social situations? (4) Does she have a
  good sense of humor? (5) Who does your child get along better
  with—younger children, same age peers, older children, or adults?
- *Practitioners and parents must realize that once a child is
  "labeled" by peers, changing this mindset in the child and the
  antagonists is a slow, difficult process.* Change must be measured
  in small increments and expectations must be realistic. For
  example, in Chloe's case, it is not likely that she will shift from the
  neglected or rejected social status to popular; but she can move to
  the accepted status over time.

SUMMARY

In summary, the cases discussed in this chapter address many of the common behavioral problems encountered in practice. These include aggression, bedtime issues, time-out refusal, toileting, homework, separation issues, refusal to comply with parental requests, and school difficulties/social problems. Most of these problems do not meet the diagnostic criteria necessary for a disorder (the exception being a possible oppositional-defiant disorder or an adjustment disorder); they do, however cause distress in the child and family, and have a potential long-range negative impact on the course of the child's development. As a result, these examples generally fall into the "problem" category. While only eight cases were delineated, the conceptualizations, techniques and general principles are applicable to a wide array of other behavioral concerns that are typical in children.

Chapter 9

Quick Reference

Signs, Reinforcements, Techniques, and Considerations

In this section, a template to conceptualize and address twenty of the most frequently encountered behavioral concerns in young children is provided. Arguably, this approach may be simplistic, but it does provide a quick reference for the practitioner. It is not meant to be exhaustive, nor does it portray detailed treatment programs such as those indicated in the previous chapter; rather this chapter is designed to offer general considerations that may be expanded upon, using the approaches mentioned previously. As was indicated in the preceding chapter, each problem behavior has its unique, as well as shared components, and this template approach is not meant to be exhaustive. Some behavioral concerns actually meet the criteria for a "disorder."

AGGRESSION (YOUNG CHILD)

Look for:

- permissive parenting.
- Modeling (by parents, siblings).
- Language impairment.
- ADHD.
- Marital discord.
- Difficult child temperamental style.
- Oppositional defiant disorder.

Possible reinforcement:

- Control (on the part of the child).
- No consequences (gets away with it).
- Behavior leads to a desired goal.

Techniques:

- Time out for negative, aggressive behavior.
- Positive reinforcement for desired behavior.
- One warning for verbal aggression/no warning for physical aggression.
- Increased "cost" to child linked to increase in aggressive behavior (step-up procedure).
- Parent behavior management counseling.

Considerations:

- If child has ADHD or language disorder, develop competencies.
- Use fading of reinforcement for appropriate behaviors over time.
- After defining and addressing top aggressive behaviors, expand program.
- Generalization should occur once parental presence (credibility) is established.

AGGRESSION (OLDER CHILD)

Look for:

- Permissive indulgent/permissive indifferent parenting.
- Peer group influences.
- Associated learning or attention problems.
- Cognitive deficits.
- Modeling in family.
- Oppositional defiant/emerging conduct disorder.
- Depression.

Possible reinforcement:

- Control (on part of child).
- Displacement of anger/frustration.
- Behavior leads to desired goal.

Techniques:

- Loss of privileges/grounding for inappropriate behavior.
- Provision of "perks" for appropriate behavior.
- Individual and/or family therapy/counseling.
- Contracting.

Considerations:

- Develop competencies in areas of deficit.
- Consideration of adjunctive pharmacotherapy if counseling is not successful (after ample course).
- Evaluate whether this problem occurs across situations.
- Authoritative parenting is desirable.

ARGUMENTATIVENESS

Look for:

- Permissive parenting (particularly if parents are high in communication dimension).
- Oppositional defiant disorder.
- Modeling.
- Excessive job demands, fatigue, depression in parent(s).

Possible reinforcement:

- Control.
- Argument is successful with the child not having to do what was requested.
- The argument and subsequent parental distress is reinforcing in and of itself, or it leads to desired goal.

Techniques:

- Extinction: Parent(s) should not argue with the child; once a decision is made regarding specific behaviors (defined a priori), it is not negotiable.
- Argument should not lead to child avoiding a consequence; similarly, it should not distract focus from the issue at hand.
- If the child engages in arguments, this may warrant additional penalties above and beyond the original infraction.

Considerations:

- Parents should not reinforce this behavior by participating in the argument.
- If arguing continues, this should warrant a consequence as well. Often this component is overlooked in the administration of the original consequence.
- Determine whether this behavior occurs in other situations (e.g., school) as well. If so, it also needs to be addressed there.

BEDWETTING

Look for:

- Family history of bedwetting.
- Determine if it is *Primary* (always has been a problem) or *Secondary* (occurs after a sustained period of no wetting).
- Clarify if this is only nocturnal, or nocturnal and diurnal.
- ADHD.
- Stress or possibly abuse.

Possible reinforcement:

- No consequences, therefore no reason to change; issue is down-played in family.
- Regression to a psychologically less stressful time.
- Control issue.

Techniques:

- Shaping and reinforcement for being dry.
- Responsibility for cleaning up/changing bedding.
- Use of absorbent pad on bed (similar to that used in hospitals).
- Use of alarm system.
- Bladder training.
- Use of baseline chart, short-term reinforcement, and long-term reinforcement.

Considerations:

- Conjoint use of DDAVP.
- Age (this is considered more problematic at age 5-years onward).
- If stress-related, then address these issues as well.

EXCESSIVE FEARS

Look for:

- Family history of anxiety or depression.
- Traumatizing incident.
- Modeling.
- Family discord.
- Excessive parental concern about child's health, exposure to danger, and concomitant reduction in maturity demands.
- Separation anxiety disorder; generalized anxiety disorder.

Possible reinforcement:

- Avoidance of situations.
- Parental attention/control.

Techniques:

- Shaping of appropriate behavior with reinforcement.
- Extinction (less attention paid to feared behavior).
- Consistency with respect to extinction.
- Provide reassurance, but not to excess.

Considerations:

- Adjustment disorder with anxious mood.
- Parents must be convinced it is in the child's best interests to not reinforce this behavior, even though it might seem harsh to employ extinction.
- Vulnerable child status.
- Could be early indicator of depression in child.
- Presence of possible reinforcing value of the child's behavior for parents.

FOOD REFUSAL

Look for:

- Model in family.
- Normal physiological anorexia (decreased need for caloric intake, 1–4 years of age).
- Permissive or authoritarian parenting.
- ADHD.
- Autonomy issues (particularly in younger children).

- Difficult or slow-to-warm up temperament.
- Symptom of underlying Oppositional-Defiant Disorder.

Possible reinforcement:

- Avoidance of disliked foods.
- Control/attention.

Techniques:

- Shaping/successive approximations.
- Premack principle (eat non-desired foods before desired foods are allowed to be consumed).
- No snacks later if meal not eaten.
- Reasonable portions should be placed on child's plate.

Considerations:

- Show parents growth charts to allay fears that child is not thriving.
- Child should not be allowed to engage in fun activities while family is sitting down for a meal.
- Family models of eating idiosyncrasies should not continue.
- Parents should realize that children will eat when they are hungry; nonetheless, they will eat junk food versus more nutritious selections if given the option.
- Mealtimes should not become a battle.

MASTURBATORY BEHAVIOR

Look for:

- Normal developmental variation.
- Isolated behavior, versus multiple sexual themes/behaviors.
- "Sophistication" in sexual behavior (e.g., inclusion of others in activity).
- Anxiety.
- Sexual abuse (particularly if behavior is indeed "sophisticated").

Possible reinforcement:

- Stimulation/physiological arousal.
- Normal developmental curiosity.
- Decrease in anxiety.
- Reenactment of activity to gain mastery/understanding (in the case of molestation/abuse).

Techniques:

- Do not punish or scold.
- Extinction/ignore.
- Remove from public area (e.g., go to room).
- If in excess and it occurs outside of the home, then reinforcement of competing response such as folding hand on desk is helpful.

Considerations:

- If this is the sole behavioral concern, the likelihood of abuse is lessened.
- If stress or abuse is the causative factor, then adjunctive counseling is recommended.
- Undue attention should not be placed on the behaviors.

MUTISM

Look for:

- Family history of similar behavior or anxiety.
- Anxiety.
- Language disorder.
- Abuse.
- Oppositionality.
- Selective mutism.
- Permissive parenting.

Possible reinforcement:

- Control.
- Avoidance of anxiety-provoking activity.
- Attention.

Techniques:

- Shaping or successive approximations with reinforcement for behaviors resembling speaking (e.g., nods, gestures, makes sounds, etc.).
- Not reinforcing the behavior with attention or putting child in control.
- Making desired activities or items contingent upon vocalizations/ verbalizations.

Considerations:

- Behaviors should not be reinforced outside of the home by school personnel, classmates, or relatives.
- Presence of actual language abilities should be determined.
- If behavior is due to anxiety, medication may be an adjunctive treatment.
- Punishment should not be employed.
- Attention given to behavior should be decreased in a firm, "matter-of-fact" manner.

NONCOMPLIANCE

Look for:

- Permissive parenting.
- Difficult child temperament.
- Oppositional-defiant disorder.
- Lack of consequences/child gets out of situation without complying with request.

Possible reinforcement:

- Control.
- Autonomy.
- Avoidance of task.
- Causing distress in parent(s), even if task is eventually completed.

Techniques:

- Reinforcement for task completion.
- Penalty for not complying with request after 1 warning.
- Additional penalty for task refusal, even if task is eventually done.
- Provision of "choices," namely, "if _____, then _____."
- Select one or two behaviors/tasks for initial program.

Considerations:

- Intra-agent and inter-agent consistency regarding consequences is critical.
- Additional penalty for noncompliance/arguing is necessary, as it does not cost the child anything to cause a conflict even if there is eventual compliance.

- Parent must not set herself/himself up by "asking" the child to do something; "telling," in a nice way, is sufficient.

REFUSAL TO TAKE MEDICATION

Look for:

- Permissive parenting style.
- Oppositional defiant disorder.
- Early adolescent issues.
- Marital discord/disagreement regarding medication.
- Too many side effects (real or perceived).
- Ridicule from peers or siblings regarding medication.
- Bad previous experience with medication (e.g., vomiting).

Possible reinforcement:

- Control.
- Perception by child that by not taking medication, he/she is not different than others.
- Avoidance without consequence.

Techniques:

- Gains positive reinforcement (coupons, privileges, access to activities) for taking medication.
- Loses privileges, coupons, etc. for non-compliance.
- Establish parental "presence," or credibility in a more general sense.

Considerations:

- Reasons for noncompliance with respect to taking medication must be identified and addressed.
- Parental attitudes toward medication must be explored.
- By no means should the child be physically forced to take the medication.

SCHOOL BEHAVIORAL PROBLEM

Look for:

- Learning disabilities.
- ADHD.
- Peer difficulties.

- Teacher-child conflict.
- Slow-learner (borderline) intelligence quotient.
- Face-saving technique.
- Control issue.
- Oppositional-defiant disorder.
- Permissive parenting style.

Possible reinforcement:

- Control of a perceived otherwise uncontrollable situation.
- Avoidance of academics that may be too difficult.
- Avoidance of ridicule by classmates.

Techniques:

- Home-school reinforcement program; selection of three to five behaviors.
- Reinforcement for bringing home note with positive teacher report.
- Consequences for not bringing home note or bringing a note that is indicative of problems that day (loss of privileges or activities).
- Reinforcements given both at home and at school.

Considerations:

- Address development of competencies in areas that are identified as problematic (e.g., academic subjects, peer interactions).
- Parents must not cover for the child; child must accept measured consequences.
- Consistency in the home-school program is mandatory.

SCHOOL REFUSAL

Look for:

- Anxiety disorder.
- Child is victim of bullying.
- Frustration due to academic difficulties that are the result of a learning disability.
- Frustration, feeling of being overwhelmed because of borderline cognitive functioning.
- Family problems (e.g., fear of divorce).
- Teacher-student conflict.

Possible reinforcement:

- Avoidance of social or academic stresses.
- Maintenance of closeness to parent.

Techniques:

- Shaping; child still goes to school, but may initially remain in library or principal's office; subsequently increasing amount of in-class time.
- Avoidance behavior is not reinforced; child not allowed to stay home or leave school to go home because of complaints.
- Child still has to meet work requirements, although these might initially be reduced.

Considerations:

- Identify secondary gain(s); address these issues via academic help, counseling, possible adjunctive use of medication.
- Parents/clinician/school need to realize that being allowed to stay home even occasionally places the child on a partial reinforcement schedule that is extremely difficult to extinguish.

SEPARATION ISSUES

Look for:

- Anxiety disorder.
- Parent conflict—detouring this through the child.
- Covert reinforcement for the dependent behavior by adults.
- Vulnerable child syndrome.
- Permissive parenting; poor limit setting.

Possible Reinforcement:

- Control.
- Overt or covert parental approval for dependent behavior.
- Avoidance of stressful situation.
- Anxiety reduction/security.

Techniques:

- Shaping/successive approximations; rewards for increasing duration and types of appropriate separation behavior.
- Extinction of parental responses to child's protests.

- Inter-agent consistency among parents; or parents and other caretakers.
- Modeling of positive separation behaviors by peers.

Considerations:

- Increase out-of-home experiences such as daycare in younger children.
- Address parent issues if there is conflict.
- Decrease parent concern regarding separation, including clarification of any medical issues or concerns.

SIBLING CONFLICT

Look for:

- Depressed or disengaged parent; sibling conflict elicits a response from an otherwise generally non-responsive parent.
- Enmeshed family.
- Oppositional defiant disorder.
- Younger sibling modeling non-acceptable behavior from older sibling.
- Closeness in age between siblings (≤ 3 years).

Possible reinforcement:

- Negative attention from parents.
- Reinforcement (satisfaction) in seeing sibling cry, lose toy, or get reprimanded by parent.
- Neither child receives negative consequence for the behavior.

Techniques:

- Consequences doled out to both siblings for conflict; conversely, reinforcement for prosocial behaviors.
- Extinction of negative attention.

Considerations:

- Parent(s) must avoid the role of "referee."
- Parents should also consider the fact that although the older child might have originally started the conflict, the younger child quickly learns to provoke the older one as well.
- Parents must not reinforce one child coming to the parent and repeatedly tattling on the sibling.

- If the parent does not witness the infraction, it often is better to have consequences for both siblings, as it does take two to cause a conflict. This differs from simply ignoring, in that neither the aggressive behavior nor the complaints has been reinforced.

SLEEP PROBLEM

Look for:

- Permissiveness.
- Spousal conflict.
- Separation issues on part of parent(s).
- Anxiety disorder.
- Vulnerable child status.
- Environmental stress (particularly with sudden onset).

Possible reinforcement:

- Child allowed to sleep in parent(s)' bed.
- Control of family in evening (e.g., by demanding parent be present when child is falling asleep).
- Parents avoid intimacy.
- Child avoids potentially fearful situation of sleeping by himself.

Techniques:

- Reinforcement (short-term and long-term) for going to bed/staying in bed.
- Loss of privileges if there is refusal to go to bed or remain there.
- Absolutely no partial reinforcement schedule should occur; child should not be allowed to sleep in parent(s)' bed at any time.
- Shaping if necessary (child sleeps on sleeping bag on floor of parent(s)' bedroom, but not in bed. This could gradually be moved closer to doorway, and so on).

Considerations:

- Parent must make a commitment to stop the behavior (use of "I'll try," is suggestive of a lack of commitment).
- Results will take some time to occur; often as much as 2 weeks.
- Other issues (e.g., marital discord, perception of vulnerable child) need to be addressed.

SOILING

Look for:

- History of lower gastrointestinal problems/difficult toilet training.
- Stressful incident (including sexual abuse).
- Onset, frequency, typical bowel habits.
- Constipation.
- Environmental reactions (family, school).

Possible reinforcement:

- Control.
- Passive-aggressive behavior (depending upon type of soiling behavior).
- Attention.
- Avoidance of responsibility/regression.

Techniques:

- Reinforcement for not soiling in pants; increased incentives for having a bowel movement on the toilet. Reinforcement should be short-term and long-term.
- Responsibility for cleaning up after an accident.
- Bowel training (sitting on toilet in morning after breakfast, in late afternoon or after dinner).
- Adjunctive use of laxatives and dietary maintenance procedures if problem is due to constipation and overflow.

Considerations:

- Medical interventions are needed if soiling is of the constipation with overflow incontinence type; if stool is well-formed and soiled underwear is left in places that would most likely be discovered, then underlying emotional causes need to be investigated.
- A viscous cycle may develop, whereby the child exercises passive, unconscious control and retains stool. After a while this impaction stretches nerve endings and the child no longer can feel the need to have a bowel movement. The soiling elicits criticism (and perhaps ridicule) from the environment, which, in turn, causes the child to retain more, and so on.
- Punishment for soiling should not be implemented.

SOMATIC CONCERNS

Look for:

- Locus of pain (e.g., if it is in form of a stomach-ache the peri-umbilical area, or, in the case of a headache it is restricted to one spot in the forehead, there is increased possibility of pain of a psychologic origin).
- Age of onset; peak age in males is 5–6 years; in females, 5–6 and 9–10 years.
- Signs of abuse.
- Secondary gains.
- Anxiety or depression.
- Family model for somatization (e.g., irritable bowel, migraines).

Possible reinforcement:

- Attention.
- Avoidance of school, peers, other activities or places the child does not like.
- Avoidance of family problems; defusing family conflicts.

Techniques:

- Extinction; downplaying attention or reaction given to complaints.
- Identification of, and focus on, secondary gains.

Considerations:

- Punishment should not be used.
- Parents must be reassuring, yet not overly focused or concerned about the complaints.
- Child should not avoid any activities or duties because of the somatic complaints.

TEMPER TANTRUMS

Look for:

- Age; autonomy issues (particularly prevalent in the 2- to 4-year age range).
- Permissive parenting.

- Modeling from household members, (preschool).
- Language, or cognitive impairment.
- Difficult child temperamental style.
- Oppositional defiant disorder.

Possible reinforcement:

- Control.
- No consequences for tantrums/misbehavior; leads to reward of some type.
- Avoidance of something disliked.

Techniques:

- Time out for negative behavior.
- Reinforcement for not demonstrating tantrums.
- Withdrawal of attention (although there will be consequences for the behavior beyond simple extinction).

Considerations:

- Develop competencies in any areas of deficit (e.g., speech/ language).
- Determine if the problem occurs across situations.
- Check on consistency of interventions.

THUMBSUCKING

Look for:

- Anxiety.
- Regressive behavior.
- Self-quieting technique (hence the need to determine when this occurs and where).
- Potential for criticism from environment; could this cause child to be ridiculed by peers?
- Stresses.

Techniques:

- Reinforcement for not engaging in behavior.
- Introduction of a competing response (e.g., folding hands on the desk).
- Coordination between home and school so that teacher can provide a cue to the child if he/she is observed sucking the thumb.

– Use of retainer-like device at night to prevent orthodontic problems.
– Extinction in that the child is not given undue attention for this behavior.

Considerations:

– Avoidance of criticism, negative attention for behavior.
– Child should want to discontinue the behavior.
– Causes of any stressor should be addressed.

WHINING

Look for:

– Secondary gain.
– Reinforcement for whining (e.g., parents give in).
– Permissive parenting.
– Slow-to-warm up or difficult child temperament.
– Sadness in the child.

Possible reinforcement:

– Attention.
– Desires are met.
– Control.

Techniques:

– Extinction; withdrawal of attention; child must leave room after one warning if whining continues.
– There is a consequence for whining above that for the associated infraction (e.g., not giving in to demands for a snack).

Considerations:

– If the child does not receive the desired object, activity, or still has to do a non-desirable task, then part of the problem is handled.
– The second component is to have attention withdrawn by indicating that if the child persists in whining, then she must leave the room.
– The third component is to have a penalty for whining if it continues.
– This type of behavior is typically maintained by partial reinforcement.

To reiterate, this chapter was designed as a quick reference to help practitioners and parents identify potential causal factors for the child's problem behaviors, flag concerns that may maintain the behaviors, and to provide a listing of techniques that can be employed to address the behavioral concerns. The behaviors should always be thought of as falling on a continuum, and that the severity of the behavioral concern will influence selection of intervention techniques.

Chapter 10

Summary and Musings

Practitioners must appreciate the complexities of parenting and the parent-child interaction. The child's behavioral concerns cannot be treated in isolation, and both parenting and child outcomes depend on three main factors: (1) parental characteristics, (2) child characteristics, and (3) the social and cultural contexts in which the child and parent interact (Belsky, 1984). All aspects of this triad must be considered by the practitioner. Developmentally appropriate parenting is highly dependent upon the parents' sensitive responsiveness to the child's needs. This responsiveness will shape the child's perception of the environment in terms of trust and optimism (vis à vis Erikson's theoretical approach outlined previously: 1963; 1964). It will also provide the child with a perception as to what role he plays in interactions with adults, and also a sense of security and a feeling of positive self-regard. There is a fine line dividing sensitive responsiveness and overindulgence, the latter being problematic and often associated with the permissive parenting style.

Similarly, the qualitative aspects of the parent-child dyad are critical because these have an impact on the quality of attachment. Attachment influences the child's early internalized representation of what should and should not occur in interactions with the environment. Concepts of the role of the parent, the child, security, and expectations regarding interpersonal interactions are determined by the quality of this attachment. Obviously, these concepts will shape later emotional and social proclivities. Extended family members and the immediate social support system will also have an impact both on parenting and the child. An amalgam of these influences (some positive, some negative, and others of a more neutral type), in conjunction with the child's own predispositions, will determine individuality. This underscores the need to establish an authoritative parenting style early on.

Unfortunately, there are multiple societal pressures that influence the child as well as the parent. Both are bombarded by messages as to what is allegedly right, what is "desirable," and what is needed to be socially acceptable. As a result, there is diminishing awareness as to what is reasonable, and what is not, this producing confusion in the parents as well as the child. Over the last 25 years there has been an increasing impact of the media on family values and attitudes. Media saturation, less time for simple family discussions, hurried lifestyles, alternative child-care, and alterations in the family structure (and a shift to more non-traditional family constellations) all contribute to the situation. There is also a greater emphasis on personal happiness and self-fulfillment, and this individualism and its related lifestyle are in contrast to the so-called conventional family (Strickland, 1997). As a result, the family is no longer a private haven, and unity among members is more difficult to maintain (Jackson & Leonetti, 2001). With this comes the realization that practitioners should not judge or blame parents, nor expect them to have all the answers simply because they are parents.

Moreover, although we have made progress in terms of accommodations for children with disabilities, there is a general, more subtle sense of intolerance for less obvious temperamental, behavioral, or cognitive diversity, with increasing pressures to achieve and conform, regardless of how appropriate or inappropriate such pressures are.

The draw toward the "mainstream" becomes evident in scenarios ranging from the need to obtain fad toys to participation in competitive sports. In the former, parents are pressured by their children who, in turn, have been targeted by commercials, to purchase items that have been hyped and which the child cannot bear to live without. The "hot toy" of the season each Christmas is an example, these including Cabbage Patch dolls, Tickle-Me-Elmo's, video game systems, Beanie Babies or Pokemon cards. More than 24 billion dollars are earmarked by corporations for commercial marketing in children below the age of 12-years. One of the implicit goals of this marketing strategy is to make the child feel that without the product he or she is a "loser." This vulnerability is particularly pronounced in younger children or those who are emotionally insecure. Parents are then faced with the "nay factor", or how long they can say no, this dependent on how often and how strongly the child pressures the parent to purchase the product. As a result, caretakers are set up by external pressures and feel that in order to be a good parent they must procure the desired item at all costs, for fear that to not do so would have a negative impact on the child's emotional state, the parent-child relationship, or make the caretaker a "bad parent." Hence the long lines, mob mentality, and behaviors that do not reflect adult social maturity. Parents need to realize that more effort should be directed toward enhancing the quality of the parent-child interaction, which in turn would bolster the child's self esteem, sense of worth, and make him less vulnerable to the materialistic pressures that he is exposed to.

Therefore, if parents truly want to participate in the "everyone has to have one" mindset, that is their option. Conversely, they should feel comfortable in not succumbing to these pressures if they perceive them to be inappropriate. If this is explained to the child beforehand in a measured way, and the quality of the parent-child relationship is good, then negative consequences will be minimal. That is to say, the child will not be devastated, the parent-child relationship will not be disrupted, and the parent will still be a "good" parent, even though the item is not purchased.

There is a similar phenomenon evolving with sports. Without doubt, participation in sports is excellent for most children, with certain caveats. There should be emphasis on having fun, children should learn skills and develop proficiencies that are appropriate to their age and skill levels, they should respect their opponents, referees, judges and umpires, and they should be guided by positive feedback when they put forth an effort. All too often at very young ages children are immersed in a sport that borders on excess in terms of the degree of competitiveness and emphasis on winning (sometimes at all costs), the negative feedback directed at them by coaches and parents, being restricted to one sport (and even one position within that sport), and endless practices and excessive numbers of games and tournaments. Once again, parents are forced into the position of feeling guilty if they do not go along with the sports zealots, because if they were to take a stand and tone down the emphasis on sports, their child would be at a perceived disadvantage when compared to other budding athletes. It is not good enough to play recreational sports anymore; rather, competitive, traveling teams are a must in order to play in high school (which in turn is an obvious prerequisite for playing in college). Parents don't realize that if as much effort were expended on academics, the likelihood of college scholarships for grades, versus sports, is actually much greater. The child is also less vulnerable to having an injury simply eradicate the entire endeavor. This also has life-long ramifications, in that academics are more likely to have a greater impact than sports on the child's future competitiveness in the job-world for the vast majority of athletes. Moreover, all too often, when sports are not fun anymore and require too much work of a high intensity, children burn out. That is why it is not unusual for children who have participated previously on competitive teams and who subsequently play extremely competitive high school athletics, do not want to continue playing sports in college. Even in earlier grades, it is not unusual for children in recreational leagues to lose interest in a sport that they are just "okay" at because of the negative feedback they receive from coaches, parents, and even other players.

Unfortunately, there are no easy answers to these difficult questions, with parents placed in the difficult position of either: (a) taking a stand and opting for the higher road to support development of the child's sense of satisfaction in achieving a personal goal, or (b) going with the flow. One should always question the parents' and even coaches' motivations for excesses in sports; that is, is this for the child or, in some other way, for the adult?

This issue has received more press coverage lately in terms of parental aggressiveness toward each other, quiet Saturdays (where parents cannot scream at their child from the sidelines), and parents signing a good-sportsmanship agreement before a child is allowed to play in a particular sports program. At young ages, emphasis needs to be placed on the effort, not necessarily on the end product of winning. There will be ample time for that later on in the child's life. Parents are also very potent models for their children, and how they behave either as a coach or spectator conveys a message to the child as well.

A third area where parents are unduly pressured involves when their child's friends' parents are permissive, while they, on the other hand, are more authoritative. This issue intensifies during adolescence, in terms of supervision, curfews, automobile use, allowances, movie viewing, and academic demands. Parents must realize that it is confusing for the older child or adolescent to see such a disparity in parenting, particularly in light of their friend having so much more freedom, independence, and "privileges." Again, the authoritative parent must take the parenting high road, and by virtue of being an authoritative parent, have discussions with their adolescent regarding the reasoning behind their actions. With younger children, this issue often involves their friends obtaining material goods instead of privileges per se.

Parents need to step back from a bad day at work, financial pressures, time pressures, and fatigue and appreciate the uniqueness of the child and marvel at her development. Great satisfaction can be garnered from helping him through crises, providing security, and being a buffer from the storms of peers, school, or the negative effects of learning disabilities, ADHD, or other disorders.

One cannot underestimate the powerful impact the parent has on the child and the fact that the child is more like the parent than peers in terms of moral values, a sense of right and wrong, and empathy and respect for others. Children and adolescents are closer to peers on more superficial, less important issues such as dress, music and language. This is why even in adverse lower socioeconomic status, inner-city environments, the presence of an adult who offers stability and a role model can deter a course of development from the draw toward gang rules and influences, and instead nurture a prosocial developmental course.

The effects of parenting are greater early on and this sets the stage for later interactions. Stated differently, there is a high front-end load. However, this is not to minimize later influences of parenting, and the malleability of behavior and attitudes to these influences. Nonetheless, if the interactional "rules" can be established early, and the parenting style resembles an authoritative, versus permissive or authoritarian type, the likelihood of problems later is decreased. While some problems still inevitably will occur, their severity will be less, and solutions should be easier.

Parents should view a child's behavior as a glass being half full instead of half empty. Stated differently, they should accentuate the positive and underscore that the child is valued, regardless of the behavior. If the parent adopts such an approach, the likelihood of a balanced, measured response to the child's misbehavior is enhanced. The child can differentiate the response to the behavior from unconditional parental regard, and therefore better accept the reprimand or consequence of his behavior, yet still feel secure and loved as a person. The ability to separate these two components may be the critical factor in parent-child interactions. In addition to the positive effects on the child, this ability also allows parents to enforce discipline, yet not feel that they are not providing nurturance and love to the child.

Becoming a parent is a decision; once this decision is made, there comes responsibility. The parent "has a life," but at the same time, must include the child. Self-righting in the child is a powerful force. If the child is valued, and develops a sense of positive self-esteem and unconditional regard, an occasional error in parental judgment will not have a major, deleterious impact on the child. Parents who are cognizant of this fact and who are reassured by it, are less immobilized by indecision. As mentioned previously, humor is a potent component of parenting and allows distance from the emotional charge, more acceptance of mistakes, and prevents interpretation of conflict from becoming a personal affront. In other words, it is emotionally healthy.

The community will have an effect on the child's behavior, and its influence increases, corresponding to increasing age. While some authors have adopted a radical stance in terms of the community, and not the parents, having the major impact on a child's behavior (e.g., Harris, 1998), this stance is not empirically supported. If the parents have not provided nurturance, guidance, and support, then the older child may resort to community influences to obtain such. However, if they have provided a strong emotional base and a sense of security early on, this influence will have far more impact. Even if there is a foray into misbehavior in adolescence (late onset externalizing problems), with positive earlier parenting the likelihood of the problem being successfully ameliorated is increased tremendously.

Parents constantly search for guidance and information to help them develop better parenting skills, resulting in efforts by organizations such as the American Academy of Pediatrics to produce consensus statements and guidance in areas such as discipline (American Academy of Pediatrics, 1998). More and more there is no clear system where the older generation helps younger parents rear children and offers transitional support. Instead, parents resort to books and the internet. The 1990 edition of *Books in Print*, listed 400 books on popular child care. In addition, there are numerous magazines devoted specifically to parenting as well. In fact, it is estimated that 60% of parents have read literature on parenting (Galinsky, 1990; Strickland, 1997).

Unfortunately, many self-help books do not take the *context* of the behavior into account and instead rely on relatively straightforward behavioral principles. Similarly, parenting groups offer general information, versus recommendations specific to a given child. Information is disseminated in a group format, and there is a tendency toward improving the skills of good parents, rather than helping parents who are struggling (Jackson & Leonetti, 2001).

In summary, Schmitt (1999) has suggested that counseling parents in the realm of pediatrics contains many components. With respect to behavioral difficulties, the practitioner must allow parents to release feelings and concerns about their child's behaviors. Second, the practitioner should provide education in terms of what is normal, and how to address behaviors that are more problematic. Reassurance, clarification, and an implicit sense of approval for positive aspects of parenting are also necessary. Finally, specific advice regarding altered parental handling of problems and environmental interventions should be offered, with the practitioner avoiding being critical and/or rigid. Practitioners should avoid "telling" the parents what to do, and instead emphasize and support the parents' own ability to solve problems. In other words, the intervention should be skill-oriented. It is in this manner that practitioners can provide the highest level of service to their young patients and their families.

References

Achenbach, T.M. (1991). *Manual for the Child Behavior Checklist 4–18 and 1991 profile.* Burlington, VT: University of Vermont, Department of Psychiatry.

Ainsworth, M.D.S. (1979). Infant-mother attachment. *American Psychologist, 34,* 932–937.

Ainsworth, M.D.S., Blehar, M., Waters, E., & Wall, S. (1978). *Patterns of attachment: A psychological study of strange situation.* Hillsdale, NJ: Lawrence Erlbaum Associates, Inc.

American Academy of Pediatrics, Committee on Psychosocial Aspects of Child and Family Health. (1998). Guidance for effective discipline. *Pediatrics, 101,* 723–728.

American Psychiatric Association. (1994). *Diagnostic and statistical manual, 4th edition (DSM-IV),* Washington, DC: American Psychiatric Association.

Aylward, G.P. (1992a). Developmental and behavioral disorders of the infant and young child: Assessment and management. In D.E. Gredanus & M.L. Wolraich (Eds.). *Behavioral Pediatrics* (pp 81–97). New York: Springer Verlag.

Aylward, G.P. (1992b). The relationship between environmental risk and developmental outcome. *Journal of Developmental and Behavioral Pediatrics, 13,* 222–229.

Aylward, G.P. (1997). *Infant and early childhood neuropsychology.* New York: Plenum.

Bandura, A. (1997). *Social learning theory.* Englewood Cliffs, NJ: Prentice Hall.

Bandura, A., Ross, D., & Ross, S. (1961). Transmission of aggression through imitation of aggressive models. *Journal of Abnormal Social Psychology, 63,* 575–582.

Baumrind, D. (1966). Effects of authoritative parental control on child behavior. *Child Development, 37,* 887–907.

Baumrind, D. (1971). Current patterns of parental authority. *Developmental Psychology Monographs, 4,* 1–98.

Baumrind, D. (1973). The development of instrumental competence through socialization. In A. Pick (Ed.). *Minnesota symposia on child psychology, Vol. 7* (pp 3–46). Minneapolis, MN: University of Minnesota.

Baumrind, D. (1975). *Early socialization and the discipline controversy.* Morristown, NJ: General Learning Press.

Baumrind, D. (1991). Parenting styles and adolescent development. In J. Brooks-Gunn, R. Lerner, & A.C. Petersen (Eds.). *The encyclopedia of adolescence* (pp 746–758). New York: Garland.

Baumrind, D. (1996). The discipline controversy revisited. *Family Relations Journal of Applied Family Study, 45,* 405–414.

Belsky, J. (1984). The determinants of parenting: A process model. *Child Development, 55,* 83–96.

Boris, N.W., Fueyo, M., & Zeanah, C.H. (1997). The clinical assessment of attachment in children under five. *Journal of the American Academy of Child and Adolescent Psychiatry, 36*, 291–293.

Bowlby, J. (1969). *Attachment and loss*. New York: Basic Books.

Brenner, V., & Fox, R.A. (1999). An empirically derived classification of parenting practices. *The Journal of Genetic Psychology, 100*, 343–356.

Budd, K.S., & Holdsworth, M.J. (1996). Issues in clinical assessment of minimal parenting competence. *Journal of Clinical Child Psychology, 25*, 2–14.

Byrd, R.S., & Weitzman, M.L. (1994). Predictors of early grade retention among children in the United States. *Pediatrics, 93*, 481–487.

Carey, W.B. (1982). Validity of parental assessments of development and behavior. *American Journal of Diseases in Children, 136*, 97.

Carey, W.B., & Jablow, M. (1997). *Understanding your child's temperament*. New York: Macmillan.

Carey, W.B., & McDevitt, S.C. (1995a). *Coping with children's temperament*. New York: Basic Books.

Carey, W.B., & McDevitt, S.C. (1995b). *Revised infant temperament questionnaire (RITQ)*. Scottsdale, AZ: Behavioral Developmental Initiatives.

Cassidy, J. (1994). Emotional regulation: Influences of attachment relationships. *Monographs of the Society for Research in Child Development, 59*, 228–249.

Chess, S., & Thomas, A. (1996). *Know your child*. New Brunswick, NJ: Jason Aronson.

Chess, S., & Thomas, A. (1999). The development of behavioral individuality. In M.D. Levine, W.B. Carey, & A.C. Crocker (Eds.). *Developmental behavioral pediatrics, 3rd edition* (pp 89–99). Philadelphia: W.B. Saunders.

Costello, E.J. (1986). Primary care pediatrics and child psychopathology: A review of diagnostic, treatment, and referral practices. *Pediatrics, 78*, 1044–1051.

Costello, E.J., & Edelbrock, C.S. (1985). Detection of psychiatric disorders in pediatric primary care: A preliminary report. *Journal of the American Academy of Child Psychiatry, 24*, 771–774.

Costello, E.J., Edelbrock, C., Costello, A.J., Dulcan, M.K., Burns, B.J., & Brent, D. (1988). Psychopathology in pediatric primary care: The new hidden morbidity. *Pediatrics, 82*, 415–424.

Darling, N., & Steinberg, L. (1993). Parenting style as a context: An integrative model. *Psychological Bulletin, 113*, 487–496.

Erikson, E.H. (1963). *Childhood and society. 2nd edition*. New York: W.W. Norton.

Erikson, E.H. (1964). *Insight and responsibility*. New York: W.W. Norton.

Eyberg, S.M. (1999). *Eyberg child behavior inventory: Professional manual*. Odessa, FL: Psychological Assessment Resources.

Forsyth, B., Leaf, P., Horwitz, S., & Leventhal, J. (1991). Refinement of the child vulnerability scale. *American Journal of Diseases in Children, 145*, 401.

Fox, R.A. (1994). *Parent behavior checklist manual*. Austin, TX: Pro-Ed.

Freud, A. (1963). The concept of developmental lines. *Psychoanalytic Study of the Child, 18*, 245–265.

Frick, P.J., & O'Brien, B.S. (1995). Conduct disorder. In R.T. Ammerman & M. Hersen (Eds.). *Handbook of child behavior therapy in the psychiatric setting* (pp 149–216). New York: John Wiley & Sons.

Galinsky, E. (1990). Raising children in the 1990's: The challenges for parents, educators, and business. *Young Children, 45*, 67–69.

Gardner, W., Kelleher, K.J., Wasserman, R., Childs, G., Nutting, P., Lillienfeldt, H., & Pajer, K. (2000). Primary care treatment of pediatric psychosocial problems: A study from pediatric research in office settings and ambulatory sentinel practice network. *Pediatrics, 106,* e44–58.

Gesell, A., Halverson, H.M., Thompson, H., Ilg, F.L., Castner, B.M., Ames, L.B., & Amatruda, C.S. (1940). *The first five years of life.* New York: Harper & Brothers.

Green, M. (1986). Vulnerable child syndrome and its variants. *Pediatrics in Review, 8,* 75–80.

Green, M., & Solnit, A.J. (1964). Reactions to the threatened loss of a child: A vulnerable child syndrome. *Pediatrics, 34,* 58–66.

Gunnar, M.R. (1990). The psychobiology of infant temperament. In J. Colombo & J. Fagan (Eds.). *Individual differences in infancy: Reliability, stability, prediction* (pp 387–409). Hillsdale, NJ: Erlbaum.

Gunnar, M.R. (1994). Psychoendocrine studies of stress in early childhood. In J. Bates & T.D. Wachs (Eds.). *Temperament: Individual differences at the interface of biology and behavior.* Washington, DC: American Psychological Association.

Halperin, J.M., McKay, K.E., & Newcorn, J.H. (2002). Development, reliability, and validity of the Children's Aggression Scale-Parent version. *Journal of the American Academy of Child and Adolescent Psychiatry, 41,* 245–252.

Harris, J.R. (1998). *The nurture assumption.* New York: Free Press.

Hirsh, D.L.O., & Russo, D.C. (1983). Behavior management. In M.D. Levine, W.B. Carey, A.C. Crocker, & R.T. Gross (Eds.). *Developmental behavioral pediatrics* (pp 1068–1099). Philadelphia: W.B. Saunders.

Hoffman, M. (1970). Moral development. In P.H. Massen (Ed.). *Carmichaels, manual of child psychology, vol. 2, 3rd edition.* New York: Wiley.

Holden, G.W., Miller, P.C., & Harris, S.D. (1999). The instrumental side of corporal punishment: Parents' reported practices and outcome expectancies. *Journal of Marriage and the Family, 61,* 908–919.

Howard, B.J. (2002). Counseling interventions for common behavioral problems. Presented at DB : PREP, An intensive review course of developmental and behavioral pediatrics. Providence, RI, August 9–13.

Jackson, R.H., & Leonetti, J. (2001). Parenting: The child in the context of the family. In C.E. Walker & M.C. Roberts (Eds.). *Handbook of clinical child psychology, 3rd edition* (pp 807–824). New York: John Wiley.

Jones, M.C. (1924). The elimination of children's fears. *Journal of Experimental Psychology, 7,* 383.

Kagan, J. (1992). Behavior, biology and the meanings of temperamental constructs. *Pediatrics, 90,* 510–513.

Kagan, J., & Snidman, N. (1991). Temperamental factors in human development. *American Psychologist, 46,* 856–862.

Kazdin, A.E. (1975). *Behavior modification in applied settings.* Homewood, IL: The Dorsey Press.

Kelleher, K.J., Childs, G.E., Wasserman, R.C., McInerney, T.K., Nutting, R.A., & Gardner, W.P. (1997). Insurance status and recognition of psychosocial problems: a report from PROS and ASPN. *Archives of Pediatric and Adolescent Medicine, 151,* 1109–1115.

Kelleher, K.J., & Wolraich, M.L. (1996). Diagnosing psychosocial problems. *Pediatrics, 97,* 899–901.

Kemper, K.J., & Kelleher, K.J. (1996). Family psychosocial screening: Instruments and techniques. *Ambulatory Child Health, 1,* 325–339.

Kendziora, K.T., & O'Leary, S.G. (1993). Dysfunctional parenting as a focus for prevention and treatment of child behavior problems. *Advances in Clinical Child Psychology, 15,* 175–206.

Klein, M. (1958). On the development of mental function. *International Journal of Psychoanalysis, 39*, 84–90.

Kohlberg, L. (1964). Development of moral character and moral ideology. In M.L. Hoffman & L.W. Hoffman (Eds.). *Review of child development research* (pp 383–431). New York: Sage Foundation.

Lachar, D., & Gruber, C.P. (2001). *Personality inventory for children. Second edition.* Los Angeles, CA: Western Psychological Service.

Leslie, L.K., & Boyce, T. (1996). The vulnerable child. *Pediatrics in Review, 9*, 323–326.

Locke, L.M., & Prinz, R.J. (2002). Measurement of parental discipline and nurturance. *Child Psychology Review, 22*, 895–929.

Loeber, R., & Stouthamer-Loeber, M. (1998). Development of juvenile aggression and violence. *American Psychologist, 53*, 242–259.

Martin, G., & Pear, J. (1996). *Behavior modification: What it is and how to do it. 5th edition.* Upper Saddle River, NJ: Prentice Hall.

McIntosh, B.J. (1989). Spoiled child syndrome. *Pediatrics, 83*, 108–115.

Medloff-Cooper, B., Carey, W.B., & McDevitt, S.C. (1995). *Early infant temperament questionnaire (EITQ).* Scottsdale, AZ: Behavioral Developmental Initiatives.

Moffitt, T.E. (1993). Adolescence-limited and life-course persistent antisocial behavior: A developmental taxonomy. *Psychological Review, 100*, 674–701.

Moffitt, T.E., Caspi, A., Dickson, N., Silva, P., & Stanton, W. (1996). Childhood-onset versus adolescent-onset antisocial conduct problems in males: Natural history from ages 3 to 18 years. *Development and Psychopathology, 8*, 399–424.

Parrish, J.M. (1999). Child behavior management. In M.D. Levine, W.B. Carey, & A.C. Crocker (Eds.). *Developmental and behavioral pediatrics, 3rd edition* (pp 767–780). Philadelphia: W.B. Saunders.

Patterson, G. (1982). *Coercive family process.* Eugene, OR: Castalia Press.

Patterson, G. (1986). Performance models for antisocial boys. *American Psychologist, 41*, 432–444.

Patterson, G.R., & Yoerger, K. (1997). A developmental model for late-onset delinquency. *Nebraska Symposium on Motivation, 44*, 119–177.

Perrin, E., West, P., & Cully, B. (1989). Is my child normal yet? Correlates of vulnerability. *Pediatrics, 83*, 355–363.

Piaget, J., & Inhelder, B. (1969). The psychology of the child. New York: Basic Books.

Porges, S.W. (1992). Vagal tone: A physiologic marker of stress vulnerability. *Pediatrics, 90*, 498–504.

Reynolds, C.R., & Kamphaus, R.W. (1992). *Behavior assessment system for children (BASC).* Circle Pines, MN: American Guidance Service.

Roderique, T.W., Polloway, E.A., Cumblad, C., Epstein, M.H., & Bursuck, W.D. (1994). Homework: A survey of policies in the United States. *Journal of Learning Disabilities, 27*, 481–487.

Rutter, M. (1995). Clinical implications of attachment concepts: Retrospect and prospect. *Journal of Child Psychiatry and Psychology, 36*, 549–571.

Sameroff, A.J., & Chandler, M.J. (1975). Reproductive risk and the continuum of caretaking casualty. In F.D. Horowitz (Ed.). *Review of child development research, vol. 4* (pp 157–243). Chicago: University of Chicago Press.

Schmitt, B.D. (1991). Discipline: Rules and consequences. *Contemporary Pediatrics*, April, 65–69.

Schmitt, B.D. (1999). Pediatric counseling. In M.D. Levine, W.B. Carey, & A.C. Crocker (Eds.). *Developmental behavioral pediatrics, 3rd edition* (pp 748–753). Philadelphia: W.B. Saunders.

Schor, E.L. (2002). Family factors that influence development and behavior. Presented at DB : PREP, An intensive review course of developmental and behavioral pediatrics. Providence, RI, August 9–13.

Shepard, L.A., & Smith, M.L. (1989). *Flunking grades: research and policies on retention.* Philadelphia: Falmer Press.

Simeonsson, R.J., & Rosenthal, S.L. (2001). Developmental theories in clinical practice. In C.E. Walker & M.C. Roberts (Eds.). *Handbook of clinical child psychology. 3rd edition* (pp 20–33). New York: John Wiley & Sons.

Skinner, B.F. (1953). *Science and human behavior.* New York: Macmillan.

Steele, H., Steele, M., & Fonagy, P. (1996). Associations among attachment classifications in mothers, fathers, and their infants. *Child Development, 67,* 541–555.

Strauss, M.A. (1994). *Beating the devil out of them: Corporal punishment in American families.* New York: Lexington.

Strickland, O. (1997). Reframing parenting in the 21st century: Does nursing have a role? *Advanced Practice Nursing, 2,* 44–50.

Thomas, A., & Chess, S. (1980). *Dynamics of psychological development.* New York: Brunner Mazel.

Thomasgard, M., & Metz, W.P. (1995). The vulnerable child syndrome revisited. *Journal of Developmental and Behavioral Pediatrics, 16,* 47–52.

Turecki, S., & Tonner, L. (1989). *The difficult child (revised).* New York: Bantam Books.

U.S. Department of Education (1992). *Fourteenth annual report to congress on the implementation of the Individuals with Disabilities Education Act.* Washington, DC: U.S. Department of Education.

Watson, J.B., & Rayner, R. (1920). Conditioned emotional reactions. *Journal of Experimental Psychology, 3,* 1.

Wolpe, J. (1958). *Psychotherapy by reciprocal inhibition.* Stanford, CA: Stanford University Press.

Wolraich, M.L., Felice, M.E., & Drotar, D. (1996). *The classification of child and adolescent mental diagnoses in primary care. Diagnostic and statistical manual for primary care (DSM-PC), child and adolescent version.* Elk Grove, IL: American Academy of Pediatrics.

Zeanah, C.H., Mammen, O K , & Lieberman, A.F. (1993). Disorders of attachment. In C.H. Zeanah (Ed.). *Handbook of infant mental health* (pp 332–349). New York: Guilford.

Index